REIKI

Learn Reiki Meditation and Cure Your Anxiety and Depression

(Learning Reiki Level 1 and 2 Symbols and Principles, Attunements, and Crystals)

Penelope Stiene

Published by Rob Miles

Penelope Stiene

All Rights Reserved

Reiki: Learn Reiki Meditation and Cure Your Anxiety and Depression (Learning Reiki Level 1 and 2 Symbols and Principles, Attunements, and Crystals)

ISBN 978-1-989990-47-6

All rights reserved. No part of this guide may be reproduced in any form without permission in writing from the publisher except in the case of brief quotations embodied in critical articles or reviews.

Legal & Disclaimer

The information contained in this book is not designed to replace or take the place of any form of medicine or professional medical advice. The information in this book has been provided for educational and entertainment purposes only.

The information contained in this book has been compiled from sources deemed reliable, and it is accurate to the best of the Author's knowledge; however, the Author cannot guarantee its accuracy and validity and cannot be held liable for any errors or omissions. Changes are periodically made to this book. You must consult your doctor or get professional medical advice before using any of the suggested remedies, techniques, or information in this book.

Upon using the information contained in this book, you agree to hold harmless the Author from and against any damages, costs, and expenses, including any legal fees potentially resulting from the application of any of the information provided by this guide. This disclaimer applies to any damages or injury caused by the use and application, whether directly or indirectly, of any advice or information presented, whether for breach of contract, tort, negligence, personal injury, criminal intent, or under any other cause of action.

You agree to accept all risks of using the information presented inside this book. You need to consult a professional medical practitioner in order to ensure you are both able and healthy enough to participate in this program.

Table of Contents

INTRODUCTION 1

CHAPTER 1: BASIC CHAKRA CONCEPTS 3

CHAPTER 2: THE HISTORY OF REIKI 12

CHAPTER 3: WHY LEARN REIKI? 17

CHAPTER 4: HOW REIKI WORKS 24

CHAPTER 5: REIKI HEALING 30

CHAPTER 6: REIKI PRINCIPLES 43

CHAPTER 7: REIKI MASS PRAYER 59

CHAPTER 8: LIVING WITHOUT ANGER 63

CHAPTER 9: THE SCIENCE BEHIND REIKI 81

CHAPTER 10: ATTUNEMENT 106

CHAPTER 11: MOTIVATE YOURSELF TO PRACTISE REIKI EVERYDAY 111

CHAPTER 12: GETTING READY FOR MEDITATION 121

CHAPTER 13: ORGINS OF REIKI (MIKAO USUI) 127

CHAPTER 14: POTENTIAL BENEFITS OF REIKI 139

CHAPTER 15: INTRODUCTION TOTREATING OTHERS 150

CHAPTER 16: THE HUMAN MICROCOSM AND THE TAOIST UNIVERSE 167

CHAPTER 17: THE VALUE OF A TREATMENT 180

CONCLUSION 183

Introduction

This book gives you an insight about a way of life – for healthy and fresh living. Yoga helps you to understand the art of maintaining the body, spirit and mind in the right track. Yoga is no science, it is just a practice.

Yoga has now been practiced for years and has proved time and again to be one of the best ways to strike a balance between our lifestyle and health, giving us stability to achieve what we intend to. Yoga gives the drive to accomplish that "something extra" which we always aim for.

Over the years yoga has gained immensely in popularity and in reach. The yogic postures are not foreign to us; unknowingly we have been doing it in our day to day life, in some way or the other. A cat stretch for backbone strengthening, or a wind-relieving position that helps in digestion process; yoga is about doing those small things that helps in a good living.

This book seeks to explain the concept and postures involved in yoga, for a beginner; it lays the path toward getting to know our boundless abilities, strength and happiness by performing yoga step by step. I want to thank you for downloading this book and hope you find you find it helpful.

Chapter 1: Basic Chakra Concepts

There are a lot of things you must know about chakras. In fact, you could fill a book with only the history of chakras, and a guide to religious people, political leaders and icons who have probably achieved balanced chakras in their lifetime. However, before you jump into the practical usage and recharging of chakras, you must first become acquainted with some basic concepts every chakra student should know. In this first chapter, you will learn about the nature of chakras, how they function, and why they must be kept in balance to achieve inner peace.

So what are these things called chakras?

The word chakra comes from the Sanskrit term which means "wheel." The ch in chakra is pronounced in the same way as the words "challenge," "cheap," or "chat."

These "wheels" are positioned in a straight line, in the middle of the body. The chakra line begins from the base of your spine, where the root chakra is located, and ends just above the crown of your head, where the thought chakra resides.

Think of these chakras as wheels, or whirlpools that sucks the energy from your environment, friends, relatives, and from your own actions and thought processes. Depending on the kind of energy you are exposed to, and the kind of energy you emanate, your chakras could either be in complete sync with each other, or become distorted and warped. That might sound frightening, and the concepts of energies being drawn and generated from your environment to your chakras may seem a little hard to believe, but as you progress through this lesson, you will better understand why chakras act as whirlpools to the never ending supply of energy around you.

Now, to further understand energy, and how this affects an individual's chakras, you must first learn a little physics. Don't worry. You won't need to learn any complicated formulas or prove any theorems for this. All you need to do is keep reading with an open mind, and try to imagine the concepts that are being presented to you.

Light and Energy: A comparison for Chakra Students.

Have you ever seen a rainbow? If you have, then you already know that the rainbow appears to us in a spectrum of seven colors. These colors, no matter how different they are from each other, actually stem from a single source of light called white light. When this white light or pure light is shined through a prism, it breaks into seven colors. Remember that though the seven colors seem very different from each other, they all come from the pure light. Each color is a form of energy that vibrates on certain levels; red has the lowest vibration, while indigo has the highest vibration. The same can be said for a person's chakras.

Pure energy, untainted by problems, illnesses, worries and fears can be thought of as the equivalent of white light. Once this energy comes into contact with a person's body, it breaks into seven pools. These seven pools are none other than the seven main chakras. The comparison between light, energy and chakras is even more expressed in the fact that each chakra emits its own color. The same seven colors of the rainbow are also the colors of the seven chakras of the human body. Imagine each chakra emitting a different color on its own, but when all chakras are opened and flowing freely, the seven colors become fused to form a single, strong ray of pure light.

Energy and Balance

The next thing you must grasp before you can understand the true nature of chakras is this: energy exists in so many forms, and is present around and within us. If you want a scientific explanation for this phenomenon, think about matter.

Recall your science lessons in high school. You must have learned about atoms, and the particles that reside within each atom. Remember the electrons, protons, and neutrons? Those particles vibrate and emit certain energy wave lengths that affect the other particles contained in the same body, or atom. In turn, the atom or containing body vibrates as well, and emits a unified energy wave length to those around it. This atom or body affects and is affected by other such bodies in its vicinity. So you see, everything, absolutely everything emits and receives energy. The air you breathe, the water you drink, the food you eat, and the people you interact with all carry energies that converge with yours.

Think about this: Have you ever been in an argument with a close friend or family member, and while in the midst of exchanging wounding words, felt yourself become physically and mentally drained even if you were just sitting or standing? These kinds of situations are examples of energy interactions at its finest. You and your family member or friend were pushing bad energy towards each other, so much so that you both received twice the amount of negative energy either of you were holding. This energy is what makes you feel bad, feel tired, exhausted even if you only engaged in verbal argument. This is energy that is out of sync, an energy imbalance that affects you as a whole, other people, and more importantly, your chakras.

Now think about this last example for to help you understand energy and balance. After arguing with someone, and refusing to come to terms with them, you undoubtedly feel burdened, and no matter how much you try to avoid thinking about the argument, it will always be at the back of your mind, bothering you. However, once you sincerely apologize and make amends with the other party, you feel that burden is lifted, and a feeling of lightness, of weightlessness comes upon you. Why? Because you and the other person concerned dealt with the negative energy, and channeled it into a more positive one. Positive energy heals the body, mind and spirit, and is what the chakras need to stay aligned and open.

The Physical, Mental and Spiritual Manifestation of Chakra Imbalances

Now that you know about light, color, energy and how these fundamental physics concepts relate with chakras, you must learn about how chakra imbalances affect us, and manifest in our daily lives.

Chakra imbalances can manifest themselves in different forms. You see, the seven main chakras are connected to seven glands located throughout the human body. If a chakra is experiencing imbalance, then the mind and body will certainly reflect that. For instance, if your sixth chakra, which can be found above and in-between a person's eyes is closed, then you will be unable to see apparitions, supernatural beings, or creatures thought to exist only in myth. This is because the sixth chakra opens the third eye of an individual, and if you never open yourself to experiences of the supernatural, then you will never be able to use your sixth chakra as well. This closed chakra point will affect how you see things, how you think, decide and speak. It will also affect other chakra points in the long run, and will thus keep you in a disharmonic state.

Another example of a physical manifestation of a chakra imbalance is when an individual has difficulty speaking or expressing him or herself. The throat area houses the fifth chakra, which controls and affects an individual's ability to recognize the importance of ethereal, internal worlds, as well as the abilities to express oneself through verbal cues, body language, art and literature. Usually, the fifth chakra experiences imbalance when an individual denies him or herself from even considering the reality of internal worlds, or when fears clog the fifth chakra from allowing the individual to full express him or herself.

Remember that chakra imbalances can occur whenever a certain chakra point is underused, overused, overcharged or undercharged.

Chapter 2: The History Of Reiki

Synopsis

In Chinese, the word "rei" literally means a mysterious atmosphere or spiritual power, and "ki" means life force, mood, power or spirit. Together they're loosely translated as "universal life-force energy." This describes Reiki, the therapeutic art made popular by a Japanese Buddhist devotee named Dr. Makao Usui in the 1920s. There he meditated to acquire knowledge and had a vision that he considered a healing art.

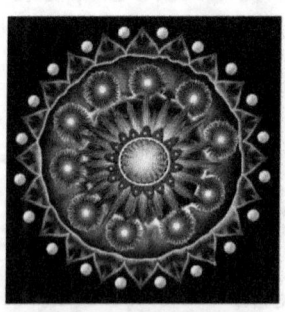

The History

Dr. Usui likewise took on 5 ethical rules that became called the Reiki healing principles, or "Goka." According to Dr. Usui, by applying these rules, which he taught, one might embark on the path towards self healing:

The secret technique of inviting great fortune into your life

The technique of using Reiki healing as a fantastic medicine for all illness

The exercise of sitting in the Gassho position (hands held palm-to-palm) and speaking the Reiki healing technique words aloud in your heart, each morning and night

The technique of centering and challenging your energy of the present day on the accompanying thoughts:

Don't be angry.

Don't worry.

Be thankful.

Work with integrity.

Be kind to other people.

Reiki isn't a religion, but a healing doctrine, and although a few consider it able to help the body heal itself, several consider it to be a "feel-good" therapy that advances relaxation.

Reiki healing treatments involve the placement of the hand on or over the body in certain places to adjust the "Chi" or life energy in the body. 12 to 20 hand positions are utilized, either touching or just above the body for 3 to 5 minutes each, and the total treatment takes from forty-five to ninety minutes.

Those who are treated report they feel warmth or tingling in the areas of treatment, with treatments being duplicated every 1 to 4 weeks.

The thought is that when the body's energy is correctly flowing and aligned, as in acupuncture and a few types of massage, the body may heal itself from a lot of ailments, as well as from the tension and anxiety that cause imbalances in wellness and health.

The higher levels of training center on treatments from a distance, with a trust that the Reiki Masters may send off energy to those who are getting treated.

The story of Reiki is blossoming even as we take a breath.

Fresh sources, adding to what we're currently being told is the 'true' history, are commonly being 'rediscovered' by investigators - though this isn't to say that we ought to necessarily trust that absolutely everything we're told are indeed 'truths'.

History in a wide sense, is at best a subjective field of study, and however unintentionally, constantly contains a little degree of bias.

The most dependable history is commonly arrived at by analyzing assorted sources - with an accent on those sources who, to coin the phrase "don't have an axe to grind", or have no true vested interest in the final result of the studies.

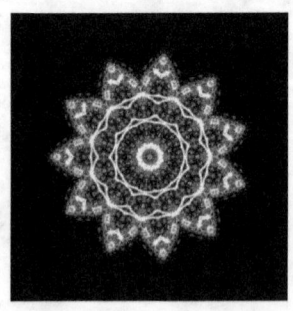

Chapter 3: Why Learn Reiki?

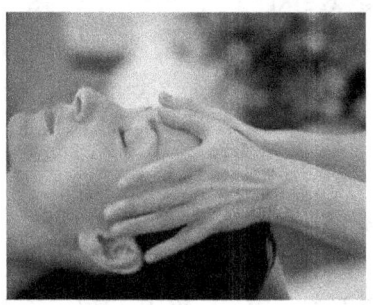

Anyone can learn Reiki, as it is not reliant on a person's intellectual capacity or a person's ability to meditate. Reiki also does not take years and years of practice. It is just passed on from the master to the student, and as soon as the process is done, the student can already perform Reiki.

Reiki is one of the purest forms of healing. There is no individual talent required or the need to develop a certain skill. Due to this, the significance of the experience will only be based on the receiver and will not be affected by the healer's personality. So, why learn Reiki? There are so many reasons why one should learn Reiki, but here are the top 10 reasons why you should:

Reiki will give you the ability to connect yourself to a universal energy which enables you to heal yourself when you need to. With its healing powers, you can balance and relax your body, clear your mind and cleanse your spirit. Spend a few minutes of your day every day to self-heal and you will see and feel the positive effects of Reiki.

Sometimes people feel like there is something missing in their lives. Something they get bothered about but just cannot pinpoint what it is. If you feel like this, chances are high that it is your spirituality you have been missing. Once you learn Reiki, you will be able to connect to your higher self, which will make you listen to your inner voice, improve your intuition, enable you to make rational decisions and feel more complete.

When your body is stressed out, it becomes more vulnerable to diseases and illnesses. Practicing Reiki has a positive impact on one's health. It can calm the body down and relax it, which provides you with a sense of peace and serenity that helps you overcome stress and prevents it from controlling your decisions, your emotions and, basically, your life. Reiki will make you realize your self-purpose and provide you with a clarity that will make you see things in a better light.

In today's modern time, it is normal to have a busy lifestyle. However, it is important to take some time off, even if just for a few minutes each day, as this hectic lifestyle takes a serious toll on our bodies, as well as other aspects of our lives, like relationships. Performing self-healing on a physical level can help prevent illnesses and relieve pain and on an emotional level can calm you down and let you think rationally without your judgment being clouded by your thoughts.

If you feel kind of lost in your own life, learning Reiki will help you remember what your true purpose in life is and will teach you how to become more focused on your goals. A lot of people spend their lives hating their jobs or their lives, but practicing Reiki can reopen their eyes to the things that they really need and make them see things from a different perspective—a perspective in which they can appreciate their life and what they have more.

Some people feel guilty about taking too much from life and giving so little in return. Taking and learning a Reiki course will not only be for your benefit but for others as well. You can use what you have learned and gained from Reiki to heal other people, and there is nothing more gratifying than the feeling of being able to help.

If you self-heal consistently and listen to your own intuition, you can expect to see your life change for the better. Your purpose in life becomes really clear to you, you know why you are doing what you are doing and you see what is really important in life. Everything around you is placed in the right perspective and you will become more appreciative of the people and things you already have in your life.

Most of us have gone through really traumatic events in our lives. While it is normal to feel devastated during those times, it is not normal to carry those emotions throughout your life, as the negative energy present during those times will always have a negative effect on your life. Traumas make people fearful and worried about the future. Some of us may be unaware that these traumas are actually the ones which have been holding us back in our lives. Learning Reiki will teach you how to let go of the negativity in your life and dissociate those traumas with your emotions. With no emotions, anxiety and fear that are controlling your life, you can feel free and finally be yourself.

It is easy to settle on what has become a customary lifestyle. A lot of people are afraid of change. Thus, some stay with the same job even if it makes them unhappy, some stick with diets that do not work, some keep on repeating the same financial mistakes, etc. If you do not become comfortable with change, these will become a cycle that may go on forever. If you are dealing with a negative cycle like this, Reiki can help. Reiki will make you see things in a different light—in a different but positive and healthy light that will improve the way you see difficulties and hardships, the way you deal with problematic situations and the way you handle relationships. With Reiki, you learn how to love yourself better and how to choose a path which will make you a happier, healthier and better person.

Reiki is a technique which attracts happiness. People who have gone through a Reiki course or treatment can really say that they feel lighter, healthier and, thus, happier. Remember, happiness is not based on wealth, on material things or on a successful career. You can only attain true happiness once you have understood and accepted your place in the universe.

Chapter 4: How Reiki Works

Imagine your daily life: from waking up to cooking dinner, from weekends at the beach to hopping into your car for work and taking your kids to school. In all these, you are constantly surrounded by what is more than the mere air you breathe and the teeming humans passing by. A dense force field of invisible vibrations cloaks you all over and has the intrinsic power to enhance your overall well-being. Reiki makes sure that you not only know but also make these energy vibrations work for your good. You must have an appreciation for these energies, that your eyes cannot see, and learn the secret of making them work to your general health advantages, and for that of others also.

The practitioner's hands act as an energy conductor of Reiki's life force energy. It is through it that it flows across the client's body—into the energy fields of areas suffering from ill health and charge them with positive energy. As soon as that is done, the part of the physical body where the negativities are contained gets the signal and begins to lose grip. All negative energies contained therein start to abate and Reiki clears the energy pathways to promote a healthy restoration.

The Reiki system is made up of five key elements. The Reiki practitioner works with these elements to get the client from a place of low vibrations (ill-health) to a position of vibrant energy (perfect health). The elements are:

precepts, also called guidelines

symbols and mantras

meditations and techniques

hands-on healing

attunements and blessings called Reiju.

These, all together work hand in hand to cleanse the body and enhance perfect restoration. At our core is a pure being— untainted and free. This pureness can often times be contaminated. Garbage— lots of it—from a low sense of self-worth, feelings of insecurity, envy, rage, depression, etc. has the propensity to subdue health and turn it miserable. We all carry it around— that garbage—in different shades, and that pure, illuminating light we all shine stays concealed beneath its sway.

You can't master how Reiki work without mastering your body make-up. The physical being you see and touch isn't what your body is all about, neither is it your spiritual being. You are your body— your total being and that is exactly what Reiki works with.

Let's get it straight up how Reiki works its magic. All the five elements aforementioned play a collaborative role. Together, they stimulate energy (Reiki) which permeates through the body. It is imperative you get to understand that the healing energy is already within you. The only problem is that it isn't flowing without restraints. The restraints are the garbage talked about earlier. They stand in the positive energy's pathways, obstruct it, and block its flow. Your resident Reiki energy flows without disruption the moment they are taken to the cleaners. It is then you feel alright and healthy—meaning the pure light of your true being is shining bright. You become free of all manners of negative contents within your being. This state is often called: "Enlightenment".

Your Reiki energy sweeps apart the garbage when conjured. When it happens, it's possible you feel it within your body because garbage sometimes plays up a bit when on the way out. That same headache might just pop up again. That stomach upset may hurl a bit of its ugly head again. You might feel a bit of tumult, emotionally. No cause for fear, you are only undergoing what is called a "cleaning process" and it is a very normal phase. It is the way of the body as it retrieves its way back to optimal functioning, pure self. The best thing to do in such times is to keep on working through it. Your body needs every support then and you must find every ethical means to provide it. That is not to say you can tolerate anything and everything. No. That would be suicidal. Stop immediately if it gets too intense or just contact your Reiki practitioner instantly.

The whole process of Reiki borders on natural healing. It is an energy that flows seamlessly within us to heal and correct— energy we cannot manipulate or direct in any way. It is all about us being open. It is about our minds letting go and allowing the greatest force of life to take the absolute reins, draw on the limitless pure energy that is offered and take what it needs for life.

Your body deserves some accolades for its everyday magic. It not only automatically takes care of all your digestion, breathing, thinking, circulation, and other vital processes without your consent, but it also possesses the outstanding abilities to self-heal. When you learn to open up your soul to the power of nature and its natural healing flow, allowing your rational mind to take the backseat, you are one with the greatest force available to mankind from the open palms of the universe.

Chapter 5: Reiki Healing

Reiki healing is catching on. The mystical power that Reiki healing has have caught on just about every adult who is into the Japanese healing art form. Who wouldn't be with the wonderful testimonials that Reiki practitioners and teachers continue to claim in Reiki-hosted websites and in books specifically on the healing power that Reiki has brought into these people's lives.

But exactly what are these people testifying about? What are these secrets of reiki healing that have changed them for the better and have convinced their friends and family members to take up a Reiki class or two?

The secrets aren't exactly a "big secret". In fact healing in Reiki is manifested instantly the moment a patient is touched with the hands of a practitioner. It is testified in the manner a practitioner lives his life before and after Reiki touched him. It is in the way he communicates with you. How softly and slowly he speaks, breathing life to every word, every phrase his mouth lets go of. It is in the life purpose he professes, that is, peace and harmony specifically harmonious relations with family members, friends, co-workers, and neighbors. It is in how healthy and fit his body is now. It is in how active and younger-looking he has become. It is in how he seems to repel illnesses and bad luck.

These and more can happen to you, too. You can have the healthiest, fittest, and sexiest body of your dreams. You can have all the good luck in the world, repel diseases, and live harmoniously with your spouse and children, with your in-laws, with your friends, and with your neighbors.

Reiki healing can make all of these things happen. Reiki will make these happen for you. This is the "big secret" that Reiki claims to possess and which it can share to those who accept the art form into their lives with all sincerity, who willfully and patiently learns the ways of Reiki, and who doesn't forget to share these "secrets" of Reiki to those in need of healing.

Start with a heart-to-heart talk with a Reiki practitioner just to reassure you that Reiki isn't some kind of cult but a way of life and of healing. Then, enroll in a basic Reiki class. Learn the ways of this ancient Japanese art form. Immerse yourself in the healing that learning Reiki should bring to your life. Savor every moment you are in a class and practice attunement on yourself and on others once you've become confident of your skills.

In no time and without you noticing it, you'll be a different person. You'll be bringing reiki healing to every person you come across in your business dealings, in the workplace, and at home. The "secrets" are finally in your hands, manifested in your way of life.

The Magical Art of Reiki Healing - A Spiritual, Emotional and Physical Awakening

Reiki is a spiritual relaxation and stress reducing technique which promotes healing, developed by Japanese master Dr. Mikao Usui in 1922. Reiki is based on the premise that life force energy flows through all of us, and indeed is the wellspring of the human life force. Reiki is performed by the laying on of hands by the practitioner.

After treatment, the patient experiences intense feelings of wellbeing, peace and security; Reiki does not treat just the body, but the whole person...emotional, spiritual and physical benefits are all noted after a reiki healing session. Reiki can never cause ill effects or be misused by the practitioner, and is helpful in conjunction with every medical technique to help with side effects and help recovery.

This unique technique is not taught in the normal sense; a reiki master transfers the ability to the student during a ceremony called an "attunement". Although recognized as spiritual, Reiki is not a religion and it does not matter one whit what you believe, or even if you believe. Reiki works regardless of whatever roadblocks we humans attempt to throw up.

While Reiki is not religious in nature, the practitioner needs to act and live in such a way as to promote peace and harmony.

The secret art of inviting happiness

The miraculous medicine of all diseases

Just for today, do not anger

Do not worry and be filled with gratitude

Devote yourself to your work. Be kind to people.

Every morning and evening, join your hands in prayer.

Pray these words to your heart

and chant these words with your mouth

Usui Reiki Treatment for the improvement of body and mind

The founder, Usui Mikao

In short, anyone can learn and practice Reiki. To dismiss it as mumbo jumbo is completely erroneous and those who take the time to investigate, study and become attuned will experience almost miraculous effects in their lives. Anyone who is seeking balance, peace of mind, physical or emotional healing, should at the very least seek out a Reiki Master for a healing session before making up their minds as to the veracity of the claims as to what Reiki does. From experience, I can tell you that it does indeed work. Masters can even perform distance healings; it is not required that the Master actually lay hands on the recipient, although it is my experience that this has the strongest physical effect on the patient.

The Art Of Crystal Healing And Reiki

The ancient practice of crystal healing relies heavily on what is called, subtle (faint or slight) energy. Subtle energy is said to be the electromagnetic or biomagnetic energy field that surrounds the body.

Sometimes, when practicing Reiki, some practitioners will incorporate the use of crystals. What they will do is lay several stones throughout different areas of the body, such as the forehead or stomach. The purpose of the stones is to release emotional, mental or spiritual blocks to well-being.

The practitioner's role is to be supportive and non-judgemental, giving you, the client, the safety to let go of any emotions and talk. This is considered to be a part of the healing process. After the stones are placed on your body during a Reiki session, you will want to pay close attention to energy that the crystals are giving off. Just as the body has it's own aura, or unique energy, crystals, such as diamonds or rubies, also have their own distinctive energy. Keep in mind that each type of stone will certainly have their own minor variations.

The traditional teachings of crystal healing have been around for centuries, and several ancient cultures such as the Egyptians, Chinese, and Native Americans have often believed in the power of crystals. They believed that certain gemstones had the ability to give protection, heal disease, and also give them a heightened sense of awareness or insight.

Many crystals have their own individual built-in energy, and will most likely take on the energy of the people or environment around them, especially if it's negative. If it's negative energy, you will certainly want to "cleanse" and clean your crystal to rid them of the harmful energy.

Three simple ways you can clean your crystals are as follows:

Sunlight: Place your crystals in the sunlight to brighten them up. Tip: Do not place an amethyst stone in the sunlight because it will cause fading.

Distilled water: Place the crystals under pure, distilled water.

Salt: Cover up the crystals with salt, and throw the salt away when you're done.

While it is very important to clean your crystals, sometimes you may have to give them a "charge." Here is how it works: Simply put, charging a crystal means adding energy to it. You may put in the energy of your crystal by applying the following technique:

Hold the crystal in your hands, and send Reiki out by picturing the Reiki symbol, Cho Ku Rei for example, and say Cho Ku Rei at least three times silently or out loud to yourself. The words Cho Ku Rei in Reiki, is used when you want to create an empowering energy.

So, if you're looking for a way to help ease your mind, body, and spirit, it might be worth looking in to include crystal healing therapy in your next Reiki session.

Thr combination of Reiki and Crystal healing produces a very powerful and amazing healing experience. Reiki which is described as the 'universal life force energy', is an ancient Japanese method of natural healing and self-improvement that uses laying of hands on a person who desires to be cured to give the experience of well-being, loving happiness as well as the gently balance life force energy. As a simple healing system, Reiki healing is perfect for relaxation, reduction of stress and promoting the fullness of Body, Mind and Spirit.

Once learned, a person will have this skill for life and can use this restoring energy to encourage equality and peace on all levels human existence. Reiki emotional healing re-activates the natural strength of your body, brings you back into balance emotionally, mentally, physically and spiritually and puts your body in the perfect condition to help heal on its own.

Reiki is strong enough to offer whatever is needed for your health but again, it can also be enhanced.

Combining Reiki and crystal healing will release a power that is potentially more powerful as both their flow of energies are enhanced.

Reiki spiritual healing will absolutely work for the greatest good of any of its recipient as it is enlightened by an endless wisdom of the world. Reiki healing comes by the channeling of positive energies that make the practitioner openly receive whatever energy the universe is sending forth. In Reiki Crystal Healing this obliges the one to be a more open channel and to possess a clearer knowledge of spiritual healing.

Crystal healing is a highly respected practice and is a healing modality that has been used since time began all over the world. Each healing crystal has different healing properties and have been known to heal a wide variety of ailments and conditions.

Promoting balance through the chakras is one of the main advantages of Reiki Spiritual Healing as Reiki and as the crystal. Reiki crystal healing will surely help the balance of energy as it is able to rush the process of healing.

The more knowledge you know about the crystal and how you can combine it with Reiki, the greater the chances of giving you an enhanced form of spiritual healing and one that will surely have higher level in all aspects.

Chapter 6: Reiki Principles

Just for today do not anger. Anger comes from a part of our brain that is called the amygdala and that I call the "primitive brain". It comes from the same part of our brain that precipitates us in fear, worry and depression. It is a useful part of our brain because its job is to keep us safe, but it becomes destructive when we let it rule our world. Most of the time, anger is only a mask for fear. And that's why the amygdala steps in. It used to be extremely useful to get angry when we lived in caves and we needed that adrenaline rush to survive and run away from bears and wild animals. However, in today's circumstances, anger is triggered all too often and usually only brings about negative outcomes. Think about how often you have said hurtful things when in anger that you have regretted afterwards. One should not suppress emotions but probably the best thing to do when you get angry is to remove yourself from the source of your anger so as not to harm someone else or yourself. Ancient wisdom teaches us that no one can make you angry, the anger is just coming out because the root is in you. The sage never blames something else, he blames himself for anger.

Have you ever noticed that some people's life circumstances are hostile and wherever they go they seem to encounter the same problem? They might go from job to job, for example, only to find the same abusive boss. Very often, these people have a lot of bottled up anger that they have not dealt with and this is reflected in their environment. And until they can understand their own responsibility for it, i.e. the fact they have some unresolved anger in them, they blame the world for their unfortunate circumstances. What Buddhism teaches us is to become aware of that repressed anger and accept it. Not to try to fight it or judge it but see it for what it is. And then work at transmuting it. **Thich Nhat Han**, a wonderful Buddhist monk that was nominated by Martin Luther King for the Nobel Prize for peace, has written a wonderful book called **Anger**, that I highly recommend, as well as all his other books.

Just for today do not worry. Worrying is the most counter productive of all activities. It comes from the same part of the brain as anger, the amygdala, a.k.a. our reptile brain. In order to keep us safe, it brings up the worse possible scenarios and thinks about it over and over and over, until it makes us sick with worry, sometimes quite literally. Worrying has never brought any solution to any problem. What it does, however, is ruin our days with negative thoughts. Let's take the example of an exam. We can worry for days on end about the outcome of it. Then on the day of the exam, we can worry about whether we are doing well and if our anxiety has reached a high level we might even have a panic attack. After the exam, we worry about how we could have done better and whether we have failed. The exam might have been one hour of our life, but we probably worried over it a good five hundred hours. Has the worrying helped with our revision? Has it helped with our performance? No, in fact it probably hindered it. So once and for all, we need to train our minds to stop to worry. To do that, we have to ask our evolved mind, the intellect, to put things in perspective and when it catches us worrying, recognise that is counterproductive and move on. Guilt is a by product of worry. It has the same negative effects and must be treated in the same way as anxiety and anger. Does guilt improve a situation? No it doesn't. And most negative emotions are similarly poisonous. Sometimes to help us think positively, we need to reprogram our minds. All these negative emotions are screens that prevent us seeing that we are loved by the great creator and that, as we trust more in that love, things will enfold as they are meant to be. It might take us a lifetime to realise this, but it is an eternal truth. Mostly we worry or fear because we fail to trust that the world is a good place to live. But also, there is a universal law that states that we get more of what we pay attention to the most. Our thoughts create our reality and we must learn to master them and master our mind to put in motion what we want, as opposed to what we don't want. Sometimes it takes such a simple change to achieve that that it seems to simple. Yet it is the truth.

There is a story that goes like this. A woman was sat on a train from London to Bristol. At Reading, another woman came and sat next to her. She was quite keen to start a conversation and one thing led to another and she told her how she was moving from Reading to Bristol. She explained to her how Reading had been really hard for her and the people had treated her really badly so she was relieved to move to a city like Bristol that seemed so much more human and friendly. At one point in the conversation, it transpired that the other woman was a Bristolian so the woman asked her what Bristol was like. She answered "pretty much as Reading is".

That Bristolian lady travelled quite a bit on the route between London to Bristol for her work and a couple of weeks later, another lady came to sit by her. That person was moving from London to Bristol. Again, she was quite keen to engage in a conversation with her and told her how she had loved London and found Londoners so easy to relate to and so friendly. She explained how she had had to move from Liverpool to London due to her work and she had really enjoyed her time there. However, she had to move again for her job. She was looking forward to the new move to Bristol. The Liverpudlian then turned to the Bristolian and asked her "what is Bristol like?" The Bristolian answered her: "Well you will find that people in Bristol are pretty much like the ones in Liverpool and London". The morale of the story is that the two ladies moved to the same city and they were going to have very different experiences which were governed by their own attitude and outlook on life as opposed to being created by the people in the city. You create your own reality with your thoughts. In fact, people react to your thoughts about them whether they are aware of them or not. This is based on instinct.

Honour your parents, elders and teachers. This is the one that we usually struggle the most with. Honour our parents. When we are young, we think we know everything. We have learnt from our parents' mistakes and we swear that we will do better. This might be true, but again, possibly not. This does not dispense us from honouring our parents, even if, and probably even more, if they have made mistakes. Life is not about avoiding making mistakes. On the contrary, mistakes, or what we think are mistakes, are here to teach us and help us in our progression. And with the right attitude, they can even be our best friends. One should not anger at one's parents mistakes or judge them too harshly. If you find it hard to do that at this point in your life, know that until you forgive them, you will not progress on your own spiritual path. Why is that? Because negative emotions hold you back. I am not telling you to rush into forgiveness. Forgiveness is a process that can take time and it can be a solitary path. Sometimes we forgive people who don't even know they have hurt us. But do we know ourselves of all the hurts we have inflicted upon others? Parenthood is one of the most trying and difficult path and Buddhism actually considers it the higher path. So if that's the only thing you do, honour your parents for having giving you a chance to come to this earth to learn. Did you know that there is actually a queue to get here, so you are fortunate to have made it?

What can also help forgive is to understand that whatever has happened to us we have chosen for ourselves at soul level for our own growth. This supposes that you keep your mind open to the idea of reincarnation. The idea, however, is that we all chose the blueprint of our lives: our parents, our siblings, our friends, our colleagues and even our enemies, or as I prefer to call them our "petty tyrants". And the reason we chose all these, despite the fact that sometimes they bring more challenges than blessings, is that we chose to learn specific lessons. Some of us have come here to learn about patience, others about forgiveness, etc.

Honouring the elders is to recognise that there is good in certain traditions and that elders are bearers of knowledge and wisdom. This was the way in Africa and for Native Americans, to name a few. Age was honoured. Since consumerism has become so prominent in the West, we now live in a culture that worships youth. In these times and ages, it is all the more important to honour the elders of our society; The ones who have walked the paths before us and often through their pains and their tribulations made it possible for us to lead the lives that we live. See the beauty in a weathered face whose many wrinkles have a story. Think of the women who fought for us to have the right to vote. Think of the men who have fought in the first and second world wars to preserve our freedom in the West. But to travel a bit further than our own country, let's be thankful for historical figures that have made this world a better place to live: Ghandi, Mandela, to name a few.

Honouring our teachers. Who are our teachers? Our teachers are often the people who anger us or aggravate us. Haven't you noticed how often these people are members of our families? This is no coincidence. When we get angry at someone, we have to stop and think: why do I get angry? Go past the first impression. Sometimes it is because that person does something that has been denied to you. Sometimes it is because they do not listen or respect us and this echoes a pain in us that has been repressed. Can we learn to do things differently? How much better would we deal with our teachers if we were creative enough to learn the lesson and move on. Try to see the annoying person at the office as a child of God, just as you are. And honour the fact that there is something good in her. Also honour her for having shown you that there is something that needs attention in you. It's difficult but so much worth the reward. I would like to suggest a profound book called the **Gentle art of blessing, by Pierre Pradervant**, to help you take this concept to the next level.

Earn your life honestly. Sometimes it seems that dishonesty pays more. In our moments of despair that's what we think. It is not for us to judge if something is fair and if dishonesty pays. However, being honest keeps your heart pure and innocent. Lies and deceit affects you on a profound level. It corrupts the soul and attracts negativity. Ultimately, you are only responsible for your own path and wouldn't you like to look back at your life and feel that you have done your best? Or if you have erred, that you have made amends? This is what responsibility is all about. It is no good saying, I did this because my parents did that, or my siblings treated me this way, etc. There might be hundreds of people who have suffered a similar situation and who do not resort to dishonesty or vengeance. The law of karma means that you will be accountable for every single one of your actions. It can seem daunting, but you will probably be the harshest judge of your own actions. And it also explains that what people do to you is their karma but how you react to it is yours. So take responsibility for your reaction to others and try to refrain from reacting in the heat of the moment. Wait a little and reflect. Then respond. Response is very different from reaction. And sometimes response is not doing anything and letting things go.

Show gratitude to all living things. Sometimes this precept is expressed as show gratitude for everything. Gratitude is a core attitude on a spiritual path. Gratitude is appreciating what you have. Suppose you have a job that you don't particularly enjoy, you should still be grateful for it because it pays you and if you lost it, you would be worse off financially. How many of us are not grateful for being healthy until we become ill. We take things for granted. Gratitude is the attitude of not taking anything for granted and of being appreciative of every little blessing. Once we can do that, we attract more into our lives because we have abundance in our hearts. How can you get more money if you don't appreciate the money you already have or if you judge money as being unspiritual? Gratitude to all living things: all living things deserve gratitude. It is not only humans. Are we grateful for the animals who enrich our lives, whether as food or as pets? And what about plants who give to us nourishment and enjoyment through food, flowers, smells, nature and sceneries? Are we really appreciative of it?

If I could conclude this chapter, despite the fact I feel this is only a brief introduction to spiritual laws, I would add two things:

☐ It is important to focus on what we want to achieve our dreams. Let's stop focusing on what could go wrong and how things might not work. Instead, let's put all our lovely energies for a positive outcome and by doing this increasing the chances of it coming to us, but always remembering when we ask to add "in divine timing and if it is for our highest good or the highest good of all". And of course never to wish for harm to come to others.

☐ It is equally as important that we stop judging others. We don't know their life circumstances and appearances can be deceiving. We all too readily judge people from what we see. Let's send blessings to all the people who come across our paths whether we like them or not. In fact, a good spiritual practice is to send reiki when you watch the news. Start with the ones who have caused chaos or harm, then send some to the victims and finish by sending prayers for those who are affected by the news and that includes the viewers.

Chapter 7: Reiki Mass Prayer

Reiki is a wonderfully beneficial system for human existence. It can take care of all mental, emotional and physical problems. But it requires Reiki attunement.

With modern ways of living and complexities of life, people find themselves at the cross roads of personal aspirations and situation constraints. People are now looking for metaphysical sources to get the required strength, power and peace to meet the challenges. Out of all the sources, Reiki is certainly the most effective one. Reiki Master Mikao Usui rediscovered it in the beginning of 18th century. The term Reiki literally means Energy. With Reiki attunements at different levels, one becomes powerful to heal anybody, anything through her/his pair of palms. The fundamental way of approaching a human system is through seven chakras located on the head through back and front side of the spine to the base of the spine. These chakras are known as Energy System, drawing energy from the Cosmic. It is believed that if this energy distribution is unbalanced or toxified, the negative impact can be felt at all levels i.e. spiritual, mental, emotional and finally physical. In today's session, let us all welcome this day with an appeal to Reiki for filling the human lives with his positive pure golden energy. Let us all feel great and pass on the same to our brothers and sisters in the world. Let us join with all our good intentions to lessen human suffering by sending Reiki healing to them.

The people with emotional and mental problems. The people with physical problems.
The people with situational and relationship problems.

"Oh! Reiki Energy! Please bless us with your pure energy". Help us lead a really meaningful life. Human life is a rare gift from God. One should be proud a possessor of this and develop a living style accordingly. Hence we all should live a Reiki way of life. In our daily life, we can use the power of Reiki. Reiki is a benevolent kind master. Our daily life can begin with Reiki bath that is sinking oneself in a vast sea of golden energy. Then feel the existence of 5 elements within ourselves i.e. Fire, Air, Earth, Sky and Water. Be in the nature and experience them distinctly. Eat very nutritive fresh and light food. Finally follow the five principles of Reiki in our every day life." Don't get angry – just for today. Don't worry - just for today. Live honestly, be thankful for the many blessings. Try to be kind to all living beings around you.

Let us heal the plants, the animals and the planet earth/Oh Planet Earth! May your Universe be filled with golden energy? May it be covered by the canopy of azure blue sky? Oh! Sky, touch the earth with love. Oh! Air, breath gently. Oh! Water; fill the earth with your loving moisture. Oh! Reiki Energy help them, help them, help them.

Chapter 8: Living Without Anger

In this chapter, I want to take the precept of "Just for today, do not anger" and look at how you can live without anger each day.

Did you know that there are over 600 words in the English language that describe emotions?

The 6 most common emotions that we experience are happiness, sadness, surprise, disgust, fear and anger.

To me, that list seems weighted in favour of less favourable emotions doesn't it?

Emotion

Why do we even need emotions? What are they for?

Well, they help us identify when our basic needs are being met (or not as the case may be), they help us figure out whether our choices and decisions feel good or bad and they identify our comfort zone and help us set boundaries.

We convey most of our emotional responses via our body language and facial expressions and this helps with interpersonal relationships and communication. Most people are able to tell if someone is happy or sad by their facial expression or the way they are carrying themselves.

Emotions give us the potential to unite as one by working together with forgiveness, compassion, empathy and cooperation. Too often though, we allow anger, fear and bitterness to divide us.

Emotions help us identify what makes us happy - so we need them!

They influence our behaviour and help us to move away from pain, fear and disgust towards pleasure and relaxation. If you never felt fear or if you never felt disgust towards something then you would never really make any changes.

It would be a very barren world if there were no emotions to feel.

It is important to note however that our emotions are often controlled by our belief system. If we believe something should disgust us then we feel that disgust.

This is clear in cases where people have been brought up to believe a certain way of life or sexuality is wrong or disgusting and they then see people through that filter, judge them according to their inner beliefs and then feel an emotion of fear or disgust towards them.

This, sadly, is very apparent in our world today.

Emotions are simply an internal reaction to an external event. You always have a choice how to feel.

Let's take a look at this choice in action by looking at a simple example: -

You are standing in a queue and someone jumps in front of you.

You have a choice how to react here.

- You can get angry and cause a scene and demand that they move and take their place at the back of the queue.

- You can calmly point out to them that there is a queue and they should move to the back.

- You can do nothing and just let it go.

How you react will depend on various factors. If you are in a rush and are feeling stressed then you are more likely to see the queue jumper as a personal attack on your rights! You may feel anger or rage and feel the need to reprimand them for their audacity.

On the other hand you may be less inclined to want a confrontation so you perhaps calmly say "Excuse me but there is a queue" and hope that they move to the back. Your anger may spike if they shrug their shoulders and say "So what?!"

On the other hand if you are not in a rush you may feel there is no point in making a big deal out of the issue and you let it go. The person maybe is only paying for petrol or something and only takes an extra second or two out of your day.

Maybe the person is rushing to the aid of a loved one in hospital and simply needs to pay for their petrol quickly - you don't know what is going on in their life.

Can you see how your emotional response depends very much on your current state of mind?

Emotions are a complex reaction based on life experience and expectations – hence the diversity of emotional responses to the same situation.

We are emotionally programmed to recognise facial expressions and body language.

From an early age, as a baby, you will have recognised emotion from the faces around you. This is part of our survival instinct. Your brain registers the body language and facial expressions that you see each day – so what are you surrounding yourself with?

If you are surrounded by a loving, happy family environment then you may find that you are more prone to similar emotions yourself whereas if you are surrounded by anger, hostility or violence then you may find it more difficult to express positive emotions such as love and joy.

The media, TV, movies, social networks and people we surround ourselves with therefore make a difference to our emotional state.

Your diet is much more than what you eat - it is also what you surround yourself with. If you find yourself constantly being quick to anger, take a look at what you are feeding your mind with.

Anger

Looking specifically at anger it is recognised that anger is an emotional state that varies in intensity from mild irritation to intense fury and rage. It can be very destructive but it is also a necessary emotion for survival as it forms part of the fight or flight response.

We tend to feel anger when someone or something fails to meet our expectations. It is often a habitual response to a certain set of circumstances.

Essentially you are choosing to feel angry.

You are probably quite cross at me for saying that right now! Nobody likes to think of themselves as choosing to be angry.

Often we will say things like "She made me angry", "I'm only cross because he did that", etc.

We try and direct the blame outward and focus externally on the situation that has provoked us but in actual fact – the anger is internal. You are choosing the angry response.

When something or someone provokes an angry feeling within you it is important to try to pause.

- Where in the body are you feeling the emotion?

- Why are you angry – what is going on that has pushed your buttons?

- What are you really angry about?

Let's put this into an easier context and look at an example: -

You have been hard at work all day and there is less than an hour until home time. Your boss comes in and dumps a mountain of work on your desk and tells you that it needs to be done before you leave.

How do you react?

Anger flares – you feel put upon and annoyed that you will be kept late at work. You perhaps feel rage that your boss is so disorganised and cares so little for your feelings. All these feelings and emotions are flying around your body – how do you react?

You ultimately have a choice – so let's look at some possible reactions.

Option A – You fly off the handle and shout at your boss, telling him that there is no way you can do this amount of work within the hour and that he is being unfair and unrealistic. Your anger gets out of control and you become aggressive and you tell your boss to stick his job (if he hasn't already fired you for your outburst!)

Option B – You say nothing and inwardly curse your boss for his behaviour. You rush through the work and don't care if you make mistakes – thinking it will serve the boss right for making you stay late. You throw the work back on his desk and leave at your normal time but then worry all night about the mistakes and have a sleepless night because you know your boss will want answers first thing in the morning.

Option C – You grudgingly accept the work and mumble to yourself about it. You stay late and do the work all the while getting angrier and angrier at your boss. By the time you get home to your family you are in a terrible mood and take out your frustrations on them.

Option D – You calmly explain to your boss that you have plans for after work so cannot stay late. You ask him to prioritise what is most urgent and you make a start on that work, promising to then deal with the remainder the next day. You also raise the issue that there is too much work for one person if staying late is the only option to get it done so perhaps a meeting needs to be held to re-organise the team or to bring in additional staff. Your assertive behaviour impresses your boss and you find that each time you stand up for yourself in this manner the better the working conditions get.

Which option do you think is the best out of the four above?

Option A isn't great – you will likely lose your job if you behave in this manner!

Options B and C are similar in that your inwardly directed anger impacts your home life after work and you affect your sleep or your family by your mood and worries.

Option D is therefore the best way to behave – however this is all just hypothetical – in the real world you need to be able to pause and reflect before you react! Something easier said than done!

Dealing with anger is a skill and one that you can learn with a little practice!

You can see from the above example that expressing your anger in a calm, assertive way is the best way forward but sometimes it is not that easy to do! You may perhaps need to suppress your anger for a moment before expressing yourself – the old chestnut "Breathe and count to 10" – it really does work!

Reiki teaches us that from an energy point of view anger rises up and constitutes a loss of control. In order to effectively deal with it and allow it to dissipate we need to focus on the hara (the energy centre at your navel) and breathe into the area. This naturally allows the rising energy to fall back down into the centre of your being and to naturally disperse. This calms the situation as the emotional response relaxes and dissipates.

I am not suggesting that you suppress your anger and hold it in – you do need to learn to express yourself – but in a healthy way.

You may find that you cannot directly express your anger towards the object of your frustration so going to the gym or out for a run may help you to vent and get it out.

Holding on to anger is like drinking poison and expecting the other person to die!

A good example of this is when you are out driving and someone cuts you up on the road. You may feel anger and start shouting and sounding your horn – road rage! The other driver is oblivious to your rage – they probably didn't even see you, which is why they pulled out in front of you in the first place. You are all full of rage and stress while they are chilled to the max in their car!

Who is your anger serving? Nobody at all!

Managing Anger

Coping with anger is a 4 step process: -

Recognise and admit that you feel angry.

Pause and identify the cause of the anger – what is going on – why are you really angry?

Consider your options.

Choose the best one and follow it through.

It is better to own your anger rather than project the blame elsewhere. For example, saying "I am feeling angry" is better than saying "You have made me angry".

Often we can use humour to diffuse a tense or angry situation – just be careful that you don't become overly sarcastic as this can then push someone else's buttons as they think you are being rude or facetious!

I often find that it is good practice to try and put the situation into perspective. I try to see it from the other person's point of view. This is another learned skill but one which is really useful for diffusing anger and frustration.

The next time someone says or does something which makes you feel angry, pause and see if you can look at the situation from their point of view. It can give you a better perspective and removes you from the middle of it – this, in turn, then allows you to come to a balanced state of mind and your reaction will be more measured as a result.

Talking is also important. Remaining calm and assertive rather than being aggressive or passive aggressive is definitely the way forward. You may also find that it is best to talk it over with an independent third party or if anger issues are really out of control, then perhaps seeking counselling for anger management may help you.

Learning to let go is one of the joys of living the Reiki way. Using the principles in meditation each day and repeating "Just for today I release anger" can be really beneficial for you.

It helps you to see the bigger picture and allows you to find a deep centre of calm to draw on when circumstances arise to push your anger button.

Placing your hands over your tummy and deeply breathing while repeating "I release anger" can really help you restore calm.

If you are Reiki attuned you may also find it beneficial to practice the art of having a Reiki shower each day to fill yourself with Reiki love and light. This naturally helps you shine your light and in turn raises your energy vibration.

As your energy vibe increases then naturally this filters out around you like a ripple and raises the vibration of those around you, making it less likely that anyone will feel the need to be angry. Win-win for all concerned!

As you learn to work with the Reiki principles you naturally become more tolerant and compassionate. Forgiveness becomes the default position and you learn to be more calm and relaxed.

This is life changing stuff – let Reiki in and make the changes you need to make. I promise you that it is definitely worth it.

Chapter 9: The Science Behind Reiki

Reiki is, in this manner, a type of vitalism — the pre-logical conviction that some profound vitality quickens the living, and is the thing that isolates living things from non-living things. The idea of vitalism was constantly a scholarly place-holder, in charge of whatever parts of science were not as of now comprehended. In any case, as science advanced, in the end we made sense of the majority of the essential elements of life, and there was just nothing left for the fundamental power to do. It, along these lines blurred from logical reasoning. We can add to that the way that nobody has had the option to give positive proof to the presence of a crucial power — it remains completely obscure to science.

Be that as it may, the disposed of science and superstition of the past is the "elective medication" of today. There are some alleged "CAM" modalities that depend on vitalism, including Reiki. Reiki, truth be told, is fundamentally the same as to therapeutic contact, another vitality mending methodology that was prevalent among medical caretakers, and despite the fact that it keeps on being utilized it is substantially less well known following multi-year old young lady (Emily Rosa) performed a rich experiment to demonstrate that it was only self-double dealing. Reiki pleasantly moved in to fill the void.

The examination on Reiki, and vitality mending when all is said in done is like that of numerous comparative modalities – those with extremely low logical credibility that is not paid attention to very by medicinal researchers. The exploration is of by and large low quality, inadequately controlled little examinations that appear to be intended to legitimize Reiki as opposed to check whether it works. The most as of late distributed investigation, for instance, see uneasiness levels and self-detailed prosperity in malignancy patients and finds that patients feel better when they get the caring consideration of a medical caretaker. The examination is totally uncontrolled, and subsequently of questionable worth. One should seriously mull over such an examination a total exercise in futility and exertion, as the outcomes were never in uncertainty.

A 2011 review of Reiki concentrates closed:

The current research doesn't permit ends in regards to the adequacy or viability of vitality recuperating. Future examinations ought to cling to existing norms of research on the viability and adequacy of treatment, and given the mind-boggling character of potential results, cross-disciplinary strategies might be significant.

To expand the extent of clinical preliminaries, psychosocial procedures ought to be considered and investigated, instead of rejected as fake treatment

Reiki (articulated ray-key) is a type of "vitality recuperating," basically the Asian variant of confidence mending or laying on of hands. Specialists accept they are moving life vitality to the patient, expanding their prosperity. The training is well known among medical caretakers, and in reality is polished by attendants at my foundation (Yale).

Reiki is a Japanese system for stress decrease and unwinding that additionally advances recuperating. And immediately one's "life power vitality" is low, at that point we are bound to become ill or feel pressure, and on the off chance that it is high, we are progressively fit for being upbeat and sound.

Reiki is in this manner a type of vitalism – the pre-logical conviction that some otherworldly vitality vitalizes the living, and is the thing that isolates living things from non-living things. The thought of vitalism was constantly a scholarly placeholder, in charge of whatever parts of science were not as of now comprehended. Be that as it may, as science advanced, in the long run we made sense of the majority of the essential elements of life and there was basically nothing left for the imperative power to do. It in this manner blurred from logical reasoning. We can add to that the way that nobody has had the option to give positive proof to the presence of a crucial power – it remains altogether obscure to science.

Be that as it may, the disposed of science and superstition of the past is the "elective prescription" of today. There are some supposed "CAM" modalities that depend on vitalism, including Reiki. Reiki, truth be told, is fundamentally the same as to therapeutic contact, another vitality mending methodology that was well known among medical caretakers, and despite the fact that it keeps on being utilized it is significantly less prominent following multi year old young lady (Emily Rosa) performed an exquisite experiment to demonstrate that it was only self-misdirection. Reiki pleasantly moved in to fill the void.

The exploration on Reiki, and vitality mending when all is said in done, is like that of numerous comparative modalities – those with exceptionally low logical credibility that are not paid attention to very by medicinal researchers. The examination is of by and large low quality, inadequately controlled little investigations that appear to be intended to legitimize Reiki as opposed to check whether it really works. The most as of late distributed examination, for instance, sees nervousness levels and self-detailed prosperity in malignant growth patient and finds, obviously, that patients feel better when they get the caring consideration of a medical caretaker. The investigation is totally uncontrolled and in this way of questionable worth. One should seriously mull over such an investigation a total exercise in futility and exertion, as the outcomes were never in uncertainty.

The current research doesn't permit ends concerning the viability or adequacy of vitality mending. Future investigations ought to hold fast to existing norms of research on the viability and adequacy of a treatment, and given the intricate character of potential results, cross-disciplinary strategies might be important. To expand the extent of clinical preliminaries, psychosocial procedures ought to be considered and investigated, as opposed to expelled as fake treatment.

As such – existing exploration is such low quality we can't reach any valuable inference from it. I dissent, notwithstanding, this essentially implies more research is required. The low believability of utilizing mystical vitality that has never been exhibited to exist by therapeutic science contends something else. Supplementary, the last sentence is odd – it proposes the creators are attempting to turn misleading impacts into genuine impacts. This is progressively the technique of elective drug advocates as it turns out to be certain that the vast majority of the modalities they support don't work any superior to fake treatment (which means they don't work).

Reiki is presently solidly in that camp. Distributed at about a similar time as the audit (and in this way excluded in the survey) is a well-planned investigation of Reiki where Reiki was contrasted with fake treatment Reiki (somebody not prepared in Reiki basically makes an insincere effort) versus normal consideration (no mediation). As anyone might expect, both the genuine Reiki and the hoax Reiki gatherings improved on self-revealed prosperity than the no mediation gathering, yet they were indistinct from one another. In this way Reiki didn't superior to fake treatment. That implies Reiki doesn't work (at any rate in the normal universe of a science-based prescription).

Reiki (articulated ray-key) is a type of "vitality recuperating," basically the Asian adaptation of confidence mending or laying on of hands. Professionals accept they are moving life vitality to the patient, expanding their prosperity. The training is mainstream among medical caretakers, and in certainty is polished by attendants at my very own organization (Yale).

Reiki is a Japanese system for stress decrease and unwinding that likewise advances recuperating.

Reiki is consequently a type of vitalism — the pre-logical conviction that some otherworldly vitality energizes the living, and is the thing that isolates living things from non-living things. The thought of vitalism was constantly a scholarly place-holder, in charge of whatever parts of science were not at present comprehended. Be that as it may, as science advanced, in the end we made sense of the majority of the essential elements of life and there was just nothing left for the fundamental power to do. It in this manner blurred from logical reasoning. We can add to that the way that nobody has had the option to give positive proof to the presence of an essential power — it remains completely obscure to science.

Be that as it may, the disposed of science and superstition of the past is the "elective prescription" of today. There are some alleged "CAM" modalities that depend on vitalism, including Reiki. Reiki, indeed, is fundamentally the same as to therapeutic contact, another vitality recuperating methodology that was prevalent among medical caretakers, and in spite of the fact that it keeps on being utilized it is substantially less well known following multi year old young lady (Emily Rosa) performed an exquisite experiment to demonstrate that it was only self-duplicity. Reiki pleasantly moved in to fill the void.

The exploration on Reiki, and vitality mending when all is said in done, is like that of numerous comparative modalities — those with exceptionally low logical believability that are not paid attention to very by restorative researchers. The exploration is of by and large low quality, ineffectively controlled little investigations that appear to be intended to legitimize Reiki instead of check whether it really works. The most as of late distributed examination, for instance, sees tension levels and self-announced prosperity in malignant growth patients and finds that patients feel better when they get the thoughtful consideration of an attendant. The examination is totally uncontrolled, and in this manner of questionable worth. One should seriously think about such an investigation a total exercise in futility and exertion, as the outcomes were never in uncertainty.

The current research doesn't permit ends with respect to the adequacy or viability of vitality mending. Future investigations ought to stick to existing norms of research on the viability and adequacy of a treatment, and given the mind boggling character of potential results, cross-disciplinary philosophies might be important. To broaden the extent of clinical preliminaries, psychosocial procedures ought to be considered and investigated, instead of expelled as fake treatment.

As it were – existing examination is such low quality we can't reach any helpful determination from it. I deviate, be that as it may, this fundamentally implies more research is required. The low credibility of utilizing otherworldly vitality that has never been shown to exist by therapeutic science contends something else. Further, the last sentence is odd – it proposes the creators are attempting to turn misleading impacts into genuine impacts. This is progressively the procedure of elective drug advocates as it turns out to be evident that the greater part of the modalities they support don't work any superior to fake treatment (which means they don't work).

Reiki is currently unequivocally in that camp. Distributed at about a similar time as the survey (and thusly excluded in the audit) is a well-planned investigation of Reiki where Reiki was contrasted with fake treatment Reiki (somebody not prepared in Reiki just makes a cursory effort) versus regular consideration (no mediation). As anyone might expect, both the genuine Reiki and the trick Reiki gatherings improved on self-revealed prosperity than the no intercession gathering, yet they were undefined from one another. In this way Reiki didn't superior to fake treatment. That implies Reiki doesn't work (at any rate in the ordinary universe of a science-based prescription).

The creators finish up:

The discoveries show that the nearness of a RN giving one-on-one help during chemotherapy was powerful in raising solace and prosperity levels, with or without an endeavored mending vitality field.

I see the creators didn't close "I can conclude that reiki doesn't work." This is odd, given that both the treatment and fake treatment gatherings had a similar impact on abstract results. With normal therapeutic mediations we close from this result the treatment doesn't work. Envision a pharmaceutical organization closing:

The discoveries demonstrate that taking a pill during chemotherapy was persuasive in raising solace and prosperity levels, with or without a functioning fixing.

In this manner – taking pills is useful. We should not worry about whether dynamic fixing has a particular physiological impact. Reiki supporters seem to have removed a page from the needle therapy handbook.

If genuine and hoax needle therapy is both superior to no intervention (they contend), than needle therapy works, regardless of whether genuine or fake treatment.

By demanding that patients must not be treated with fake treatments like Reiki, researchers likewise advocate that they get medications that work better that fake treatment. For example, rub has been appeared to improve the prosperity of malignant growth patients past a misleading impact. On the off chance that a patient gets a back rub with compassion, compassion, time, comprehension and devotion, she would profit by the misleading impact — simply like the Reiki persistent — at the same time, moreover, she would likewise profit by the particular impact of the treatment that back rub does and Reiki doesn't offer.

This is a basic point that I have been making moreover. You can't legitimize inadequate medicines essentially because they give a misleading impact. That is because viable medications additionally give a similar misleading impact, yet also give explicit advantages since they really work.

I would contend that there are additionally numerous potential damages from persuading patients that informal medicines are compelling a result of their vague misleading impacts. This is a duplicity, disregards understanding self-governance and educated assent, and sets them up to maybe depend on inadequate "otherworldly" medicines for non-self-restricting sicknesses.

Altogether, for doctors and other social insurance experts to suggest a treatment or mending practice to patients, they need proof that it is protected and effective.

About security, there have been no detailed negative impacts from Reiki in any of the exploration studies. This is reasonable given that no substance is ingested or connected to the skin, and Reiki contact is non-manipulative (and can be offered off the body when required).

Is Reiki viable?

That leaves the inquiry: is Reiki viable? Or on the other hand, more absolutely, from an exploration point of view, what is Reiki viable for?

A Reiki expert would respond to that question by saying, "Reiki is successful for reestablishing harmony, which can appear in various ways, contingent upon the ebb and flow need of the person." That's not an answer that interests to therapeutic analysts, who are accustomed to reading medications for explicit sicknesses instead of medicines to advance health or reestablish harmony.

Regarded restorative research is intended to address quite certain inquiries. Albeit regular drug has since quite a while ago incorporated an idea of homeostasis, or fundamental equalization, there has generally been no unmistakable meaning of this idea that can be utilized to test the theory that Reiki advances balance. Given the unclearness of the term pressure and the distinctions in human bodies and the conditions in which they live and work, how might science measure a person's parity?

What results have been contemplated?

Until now, the essential results examined in Reiki research have utilized measures for torment, uneasiness, and stress, including pulse, circulatory strain, salivary cortisol, just as measures for occupation burnout and minding adequacy. Increasingly explicit measures have been utilized to assess results for stroke recovery, despondency, and other ceaseless wellbeing conditions. Given the moderately unpretentious and complex nature of Reiki practice, these measures may not sufficiently catch the lived understanding of those getting Reiki. Measures that join personal satisfaction, quiet fulfillment, and stress decrease may have the best potential for showing the advantages of Reiki practice.

What is a portion of different issues in inquiring about Reiki?

Examining modalities, for example, Reiki raises different inquiries.

Unsatisfactory quality of randomized controlled preliminaries

The randomized controlled preliminary is appropriate to contemplating the effect of pharmaceutical items (albeit ongoing improvements have demonstrated that even this line of request can be controlled).

In any case, is the straight straightforwardness of the randomized controlled preliminary appropriate to considering treatments that unmistakably inspire complex, multileveled, quick and enduring reactions, for example, is seen with Reiki? Many regarded specialists think not, and a discourse about how best to examine Reiki and other integrative treatments and mending practices has started. Frameworks hypothesis is progressively observed as giving an increasingly suitable way to deal with concentrate the snare of connections engaged with integrative treatments. Subjective research may likewise give a more extensive focal point in producing important information. An exceptional perplexing variable in Reiki research is controlling for the impacts of human touch. Do Reiki beneficiaries have improved results since they have gotten continued human touch? Moreover, how would you make a fake treatment standard for a hands-on mending strategy? In 1999, fake treatment institutionalization was brought into Reiki investigate, exhibiting that review members couldn't separate between the personality of fake treatment and Reiki experts. The expansion of a fake treatment arm in Reiki research fortifies investigation structure and addresses the perplexing variable of human touch. Powerlessness to archive the biofield. Another obstruction to Reiki research is the powerlessness of contemporary innovation to record the presence of the biofield, considerably less investigation its cosmetics or measure changes in it. Superconducting quantum impedance gadgets (SQUIDs) measure incredibly little attractive fields and may later on demonstrate helpful to this investigation. The speed with which mechanical advances are being made may imply that the required innovation is on the very edge of improvement. Nonetheless, it is additionally conceivable that Reiki or biofields lie outside the bioelectromagnetic range. Luckily, it isn't important for science to record the presence of either Reiki or the biofield so as to gauge the effect of Reiki on the human framework (headache medicine was utilized for a long time before science started to see how it functions). Albeit a few impacts of Reiki are quantifiable, for example, improved pulse and circulatory strain, numerous normally detailed advantages of rehashed Reiki sessions, for example, a feeling of profound association and upgraded confidence, may not be quantifiable. It is as yet critical to archive these detailed advantages.

Patients who feel all the more profoundly associated and who just rest easy thinking about themselves likely could be patients who are simpler to treat and who are better prepared to pursue treatment conventions. Along these lines, Reiki may be appeared to fundamentally, yet in a roundabout way, sway therapeutic results by supporting the capacity of patients to get to ordinary prescription and increase an elevated attention to their very own needs.

What is the status of the exploration?

While the discussion on how best to think about integrative treatments, for example, Reiki is picking up steam, explore endeavors have been and keep on being made. In any case, investigation into Reiki is simply starting.

Other distributed investigations have taken a gander at the impact of Reiki on proportions of pressure hormones, pulse, pulse, and insusceptible responsivity, and on emotional reports of anxiety, torment and depression. The investigations to date are normally little, and only one out of every odd examination is all around structured. Notwithstanding, covering information from a portion of the more grounded examinations bolster the capacity of Reiki to decrease uneasiness and torment, and propose its convenience to prompt unwinding, improve weakness and burdensome side effects, and fortify generally prosperity. The Cochrane Database of Systematic Reviews contains an audit on the utilization of touch treatments (counting Reiki) for torment and a convention for utilization of Reiki for mental side effects.

Reiki has been progressively offered as a component of work environment wellbeing projects to address burnout and improve abilities in medicinal services and different enterprises, too as in college health focuses.

Chapter 10: Attunement

What is an Attunement?

What happens during Attunement?

To be able to work with Reiki one need to receive an **attunement** from a qualified Reiki Master - this can be received in person or distantly (online) as energy has no restriction of time and distance. The Reiki energy remains the same but the way of teaching differs from one master to the other.

What is an Attunement?

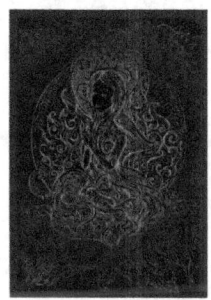

Attunement - a feeling of being "at one" with all.

An attunement is awareness of our hidden power. It's a beautiful spiritual experience by which a person receives the ability to transmit Reiki energy; this experience could vary from person to person. Attunement is a traditional spiritual procedure that helps us to connect to Higher Energy Source.

An attunement lasts for a lifetime, if you stop practising Reiki due to any reasons, no need to worry. You can start it up immediately whenever your get comfortable even after few days, months or years. Once you are attuned by a Reiki master, Reiki healing energy will automatically start flowing through your body.

Reiki energy is passed on from teacher to the student. If one becomes a Reiki master then she/he will be the part of series of teachers leading back to the founder of the Reiki system one is practising. In Usui Reiki, the lineage would lead back to Dr. Mikao Usui.

What happens during Attunement?

At the time of attunement, students need to close their eyes so they can easily focus on what they are experiencing. During the initiation, the Reiki Master activates the ancient symbols and mantras. Reiki energy flows through the Reiki master and passes onto the student. It makes required adjustments in the student's energy pathways, opens chakras and connects to the Reiki source. At the time of attunement the Reiki Master opens the main energy channel of the student and allows universal energy to flow more freely and deeply into the student's body.

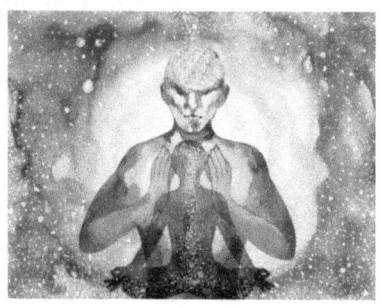

During the attunement, some students feel warmth in the hands; some may see colors, bright lights and some may just feel relaxed. Reiki works on its own intellect; it adjusts itself exactly in the right way for each student. It heals the blockages and helps to receive higher divine grace and knowledge as per ones Karma.

Once you get attuned from a Reiki Master, practice Reiki "**every day**". From day **1** to day **21** it's compulsory to practice continuously without fail, as 21 is a sacred number which signifies initiation, transformation and mastery. 21also represent the number of pathways of energy in the "Tree of Life".

Chapter 11: Motivate Yourself To Practise Reiki Everyday

By Haripriya Suraj

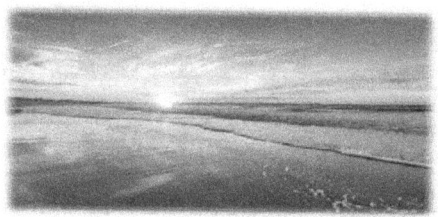

A client of mine who is also a Reiki practitioner expressed her frustration at not being able to keep up with Reiki practice. And she is not the first one facing this issue. It would not be an exaggeration to say that at least 80% (possibly even more) of people who are attuned to Reiki do not practise daily self-healing. Have you ever wondered why this is so? What goes wrong midway? Why do people lose the motivation to practise? The same people who are thrilled about getting a Reiki attunement and becoming Reiki healers lose their enthusiasm. They begin to treat daily self-healing as yet another task to accomplish.

The root cause of this widespread problem in the Reiki community is a lack of understanding about how Reiki works.

Reiki is not a magic pill. It is a way of life. Why do we brush our teeth and take a shower? We don't need a reason to brush and shower. So is it with Reiki. We do not practise Reiki because we want to witness miracles every day. We practise it because it is meant to be practised every day. A Reiki self-healing is like a shower for the energy body.

The occurrence of miracles is a by product of Reiki practice and not the goal. Soul mates may not appear within a week of practice. Illnesses do not disappear with one healing session. And life does not transform into an unbelievable miracle overnight. A lot of people come into Reiki practice with such hopes and tend to believe that Reiki will solve all their problems in a jiffy. However, it is not Reiki's job to create miracles for us. It is our job. If this is not understood, people lose the will to practise. Even when someone says they cannot find the time to practise, the underlying reason is that Reiki did not live up to their misconstrued expectations. If Reiki could indeed create miracles everyday while we sat back and did nothing, even the busiest and laziest among us would find the time and energy to practise!

This is not to discount the blessings that Reiki brings us. Reiki does bring us amazing blessings. It can help us find our soul mates, heal our illnesses and transform our difficulties into opportunities. But notice the wording: Reiki can help US. We need to do our homework too, which means we take responsibility for our lives.

And the moment we take responsibility, Reiki helps us create miraculous and purposeful lives. It does this by helping us shake off toxic energies and stepping up our vibration. When our energies are clean and pure, we experience more power and freedom. We become masters of our destinies. Expecting Reiki to do all the work, while we sit back and relax, just does not help.

The best way to allow Reiki to help us is to practise daily self-healing. A small shift in perspective will help us see that daily self-healing is not such a difficult task after all. We do not have to fast or do penance. We are not required to do complicated rituals or difficult meditation practices. All that is required is that we relax for about forty minutes and bask in a cocoon of warm healing energy (with soothing music and aromatic incense if you please). It is like indulging in a divine spa therapy in the comfort of home every day! How much easier can things get? Think about it.

We owe this time for daily self-healing to ourselves. Life is not about always rushing around to get things accomplished, meeting everyone's needs but our own and not having even a moment to ourselves. In fact, it is quite the opposite. The more quality time we give ourselves, the more everyone around us benefits too. When we are committed to daily Reiki practice, we are high in energy and spirit. We have more love to share, more joy to spread and more miracles to create. We may face challenges along the way, but we also acquire the power to turn each of our challenges into opportunities for growth.

My dear friends do hurry up and fasten your seat belts! You don't want to waste a moment more. You signed up for this exciting journey and also got your ticket during the attunement. So, what are you waiting for? Board the plane to Reiki Land and fly high!

10 Ways to Fit Self Reiki into Your Day

By Angie Webster

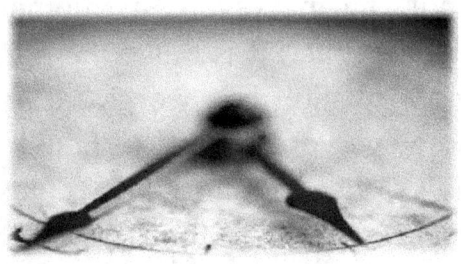

One of the biggest things I see as a comment from other Reiki practitioners is that they can't find time to do daily self-Reiki. Some say they don't do self Reiki at all because they don't have time. Schedules are demanding, for sure. So I wanted to make a list of 10 ways that might spark the imagination and get folks thinking of creative ways to fit the wonderful gift of self Reiki into their day, if only for a minute or two here and there. It makes such a difference!

1. **Do self-Reiki as you fall asleep at night.** No need to make it complicated. Simply place your hands wherever you feel led to that night and ask Reiki to flow. Allow yourself to drift off to sleep like this. Not only do many people find this a simple way to fit Reiki into their day, it is an amazing way to fall asleep!

2. **Set an alarm to do self-Reiki for a few minutes when you first wake up in the morning.** Some people find they are more able to fit this in and it is a refreshing and relaxing way to start the day. You could make it part of a meditation routine, if you have one.

3. Give yourself Reiki as you browse the Internet.

4. **Watching TV or a movie is a very good time to do self-Reiki.** Take advantage of the fact that you are sitting still and relaxing to increase the relaxation.

5. **While you are waiting in line.** Waiting in lines challenges our patience. So take the opportunity to strengthen yourself. Any line works. The bank, the take out place, a long line in traffic. Just one hand placed discreetly on yourself keeps you calm and gives you a dose of self-Reiki.

6. One of my personal favorites is **while cuddling with someone**. I place on hand on the person I am cuddling and one hand on myself and let the Reiki flow. We make a big Reiki healing loop and everyone benefits.

7. Place one hand over each chakra for 3-5 deep breaths as you let Reiki flow. Do this as often as you have time.

8. **If you find you have no free hands and you still want to do a bit of self-Reiki, you can simply ask Reiki to flow into you!** If you are attuned, Reiki is already flowing through you. Ask for it to flow and notice how you feel in the top of your head, your heart and your hands and feet. You may not always notice much, but very often you will feel tingling and warmth in these areas.

9. **Give yourself Reiki while you read!** Whether it's a great story, a magazine, a textbook, or something online(even this article--hint, hint!),while you're reading is a great time to place a hand on yourself for Reiki.

10. **While outdoors in nature.** This is a favorite time for me to take self Reiki. There are many ways to do it. Ask Reiki to flow as you walk. Sit under a tree and give yourself Reiki or simply ask it to flow. You may feel the energy of the tree, as well.

Lay on the ground and do self Reiki, if you have time. I highly recommend doing this at least once. It is an amazing experience. Highly grounding and full of wonderful energy. Very healing.

Remember, the effects of Reiki are cumulative and its effects are often subtle! You have to keep doing it to see the biggest results, but the results are amazing in the long haul!

Chapter 12: Getting Ready For Meditation

Since you already know how to sit from the previous chapter, you will also use this sitting position for your meditation practice. What you won't be accustomed to is thinking of nothing. After all, we are encouraged to use our minds and sometimes the mind becomes so cluttered with thoughts that we cannot find a way forward. You can't find peace because you have none inside of your mind, and that's where meditation comes in. This is a series of breathing exercises and coupling those exercises with thinking of nothing.

Experiment in thought

Close your eyes for a few moments and try to think of nothing. See how long you last. The chances are that you won't last long at all before thoughts start to pop into your head. There was a very good explanation of this in a book by Elizabeth Gilbert. She was visiting an Ashram and was trying to find inner peace, following a sticky divorce. What she found and what you will probably find is that you fight that emptiness. It's alien to you and your mind starts to do somersaults rather than face up to thinking of nothing. When I read of her experience and the inner turmoil that she experienced, it reminded me of when I learned meditation and I experienced the exact same thing.

Time yourself and see how long you can last. It won't be that long and your mind will fight as our minds did because thinking of nothing is alien to human beings.

Giving the mind something to concentrate on

When you want to keep a child quiet, you give it something to concentrate on in the hope that the child will be entertained. In the case of yoga meditation, it is your mind that needs to be entertained, but you also need to know that you are breathing in the correct way. The idea of this exercise is to give your mind something to concentrate on other than the daily thoughts that you have. Meditation is a time when you are to think of absolutely nothing except that which is specified. In Hatha meditation, you concentrate on your breathing. Thus, try to close your eyes and imagine breath as a thing, rather than something abstract. Imagine that you can see it coursing through your body. Think of it as energy, just like you would with flames. Feel the air going through your body, see it, feel it, hold it for a moment and then feel the release of that air from your body. All that you are concentrating on is that air mass. At the end of an inhale and exhale, count to one and progressively all the way to ten. Thus:

Inhale – exhale – one

Inhale – exhale – two

Inhale – exhale – three

Etc. until you reach ten. Then you start back at one again. If you find that thoughts enter your head, start back at one again until you can continually do this without letting thoughts enter your head. That's all there is to meditation. You may not appreciate it at this moment in time but what you are doing is tidying up all those boxes of thoughts and not letting them interrupt your flow of peace and tranquility. It takes a bit of practice to get it right and you may even need to practice relaxation techniques to get you there, but once you can see the air as something tangible and imagine it going into your body and out of your body without interruption of thought, then you are indeed meditating.

How meditation helps you

Meditation helps you in several ways, but the biggest from my point of view is that it rests the mind. When the mind is rested, what happens is that the subconscious is able to work as it should and can help you come up with all kinds of solutions to life's problems. You feel at peace with yourself and your blood pressure goes down. The flow of hormones through your body is healthier and you actually feel refreshed and very happy at the end of a very successful session of meditation. It helps you to concentrate, to be more single minded. It helps you to be able to take time and not make rash decisions and above all, it helps you to become very positive in your approach to life.

This should be practiced every day, even if you can only manage fifteen minutes a day to start off with. Do it at a time when you are totally relaxed and will not be interrupted and avoid doing it immediately after eating. When you have finished your session, take your time to get back into the rhythm of your life because this will give you maximum benefit. When you are more experienced at meditation, you will be able to do this for longer lengths of time and be able to glean all of the benefits of meditation, though for now, be content with the effort that you have made. I use meditation either first thing in the morning with the sunrise or in the early evening but you can choose a time when you are at your most relaxed.

Chapter 13: Orgins Of Reiki (Mikao Usui)

HISTORY OF HEALING

Why is it important to understand the history of Reiki (and other forms of healing)?

It is important for many reasons, including understanding the role of Mikao Usui, the lineage and how Reiki has developed over the past 100 years.

It is also important to understand that there are other types of Reiki and healing, so it is difficult to say the exact history and origin of healing. This includes healing throughout different cultures and ages, such as: -

- Ancient Egypt and Babylon (e.g. Imhotep and Priest of Aesculapius),

- Ancient Greece (Pythagoras, Hippocrates (460-377 BC),

- Cave men (shown by wall paintings in the caves),

- The Old Testament (1 Kings Chapter 17 verses 7-24, the prophet Elijah; Prophet Elisha 2 Kings Chapter 4 verses 18-37),

- The New Testament (Jesus), Jewish (a sect called the Essences),

- Faith healing,

- Shamanism ('laying on of hands'),

- Pagan times (the Priest would heal the sick)

- Kings and Queens in France and Britain (When monarchs were held to rule by Divine right, it was believed that touching them with a coin and then wearing it was a cure for ailments. A `Touching Ceremony' first took place in the reign of Edward the Confessor and last in the reign of Queen Anne. The practice of 'royal healing' reached its peak at the end of the

17th century when Charles II was giving the 'royal touch' to around five thousand sufferers a year).

- And many more.

As far as Reiki today is concerned, generally, we use Mikao Usui as a starting point. The rest of this chapter looks at useful background history, including Mikao Usui.

SUMMARY OF REIKI HISTORY

Below is a summary of the history of Reiki. You do not need to memorise this. Some of this is taken from the full William Lee Rand article featured in this book. There are other articles and up-to-date research.

MIKAO USUI

- Mikao Usui (also known as Usui Sensei) was born 15th August 1865 in Taniai, near Nagoya, Japaninto a family that had practiced Zen Buddhism for many generations.

- He was ill with Cholera and had a spiritual experience when close to death in hospital.

- He is sometimes referred to as Dr. Usui but I believe that he was not a Doctor although studied health, medical science, history, psychology, religion, ancient Sanskrit, sutras, divination and healing (including ancient methods of hands on healing). He travelled to Europe, America and studied in China. He also studied the Japanese version of Chi Kung called Kiko.

- He noticed that the healing techniques that he was studied depleted the energy of the healer (they were not channeling energy from another source but using their own).

- March 1922, Usui Sensei was meditating again on Mount Kurama on a 21-day course with Tendai Buddhist Temple because of problems in his personal and professional life. During one practice, he was filled with Reiki energy and saw the same symbols that he had read in the ancient Sanskrit sutras.

- Afterwards, he stubbed his toe. When he accidentally began healing it with his hands. He ate a healthy meal even though he had just fasted for 21 days. He healed the woman who served him the food who had toothache. He also healed his monastery friend who he found in bed with severe arthritis. These are known as the four miracles. Usui Sensei realised he had discovered healing (the wisdom and practice to actually use the ancient methods in the sutras). He called it Reiki.

- He practiced this Reiki on his family. He developed it further (Shin-Shin Kai-Zen Usui Reiki Ryo-Ho and Usui Reiki Ryoho) using experience and previous study (religious practices, philosophy, and spiritual disciplines).

- He went on to heal some beggers but they choose to still beg as they said it was an easier way of life. Unhappy, Usui meditated once more and found the five principles.

- April 1922, Usui moved to Tokyo to open a Reiki clinic and form a society called Usui Reiki Ryoho Gakkai. He taught and gave treatments.

- In 1923, an earthquake in Tokyo killed approximately 1400 people and injured many. Usui used Reiki on them.

- He travelled to Kure, Hiroshima, Osaka, Fukuyama to share Reiki.

- 9th March 1926, Usui Sensei died from a stroke whilst travelling. His grave is said to be at Temple at Suginami Tokyo, but some claim that his ashes are scattered elsewhere.

- In his life he taught approximately 2,000 students. He initiated 20 master teachers including Chujiro Hayashi (although, J. Ushida was the successor to Usui Sensei, not Hayashi).

CHUJIRO HAYASHI

- In 1925, aged 47, Chujiro Hayashi trained with Usui Sensei to learn Reiki.

- He later left the Usui society and started his own Reiki practice Reiki Ryoho. This was based more on physical, medical experience as he was a doctor in the Navy (graduated Dec 1902).

- He created medical notes.

- He wrote the Reiki Ryoho Hoshin Shishin manual (Guidelines For Reiki Healing Method), based on medical notes on which hand positions suit which ailments.

- Hayashi also introduced treating a client whilst they were lay down on a treatment table, rather than in a chair.

- He changed the attunement process and training techniques.

- He introduced healing from several practitioners at the same time, rather than one person (similar to Reiki Shares or Reiki Groups).

- 1937, he travelled to Hawaii prior to World War 2 (including Pearl Habour attack 7 December 1941). He was later asked to provide information as an ex-military man such as warehouse locations in Honolulu. He refused and was declared a traitor by Japan.

- Therefore, 11 May 1940, aged 59 he died of ritual suicide in meditation called Seppuku.

- One of his students included Mrs. Hawayo Takata.

MRS HAWAYO TAKATA

- Born 24 December 1900 at Kauai, Hawaii.

- October 1930, her husband died aged 34 which meant she had 5 years of hard labour in the sugar cane fields. This led to a lung condition, abdominal pain and a nervous breakdown. Shortly after one of her sister's died so Mrs Takata travelled back to Japan to give her parents the news.

- Whilst in Japan, she was told in hospital that she had a tumour, asthma, gallstones and appendicitis. She visited Hayashi's clinic instead of surgery, then worked with him for one year until becoming a master on 21st Feb 1938 (13 masters in total).

- During 1937, Mrs. Hawayo Takata introduced Reiki to the West. She trained many Reiki practitioners in her clinics in Hawaii, but didn't train any Reiki Masters until after 1970, and charged a large training fee.

- She said that all other Reiki Masters in Japan had died during World War 2. This was later found to be not true with the society founded by Usui still existing today. Master taught by Takata were told not to research or encourage others to research as their knowledge and training was complete.

- She believed students should have one teacher and removed the manuals and written notes – everything was verbal. I personally feel that she may have been partly influenced by poverty she had experienced in her life, particularly as a single woman caring for a family.

- She taught Reiki different to both Usui and Hayashi. She simplified and standardised the hand positions so that they were all the same (The Foundation Treatment of 8 positions). She eliminated Japanese Reiki Techniques.

- Symbols were more important in the Hayashi-Takata lineage.

- She is credited with making Reiki popular in the West. She initiated 22 Reiki Masters.

- 11 December 1980, she died just before her 80th birthday.

IRIS ISHIKURA

- Iris Ishikura had become a Reiki Master under Hawayo Takata. She also studied with different Reiki teachers. She trained two Reiki Masters but charged a normal fee, rather than expensive. She made her students carry on this fee tradition and also introduced workbooks, notes and tape recordings.

- Reiki has since grown throughout the world. Different practices have been set established. I have included some of these practices and Reiki schools in Chapter 20 at the end of this book, for reference purposes.

OTHER SCHOOLS E.G. WILLIAM LEE RAND

- This book and my school, Reiki Healing, attempts to simplify and bring these practices together (and Spiritual Healing). I have a great deal of respect for the other individual practices, including Reiki Schools set up by William Lee Rand.

Chapter 14: Potential Benefits Of Reiki

"At the point when the stream of the "Life Force Energy" is disturbed, debilitated or blocked, passionate or wellbeing issues have a tendency to happen. Lopsided characteristics can be brought about from numerous circumstances happening in our lives, for example, enthusiastic or physical injury, harm, negative musings and sentiments, including trepidation, stress, uncertainty, outrage, tension, negative self-talk, lethality, dietary exhaustion, damaging way of life and connections, disregard of self and absence of adoration for oneself or others, from feelings that are not communicated in a solid manner"

Reiki is phenomenal for mending any physical, mental, passionate and otherworldly issues of any sort and it gives grand results.

Reiki is a recuperating craftsmanship in view of the enthusiastic vibration of the human body.

Every part of the human body is a vibration communicated as a shading or mass of vitality.

Reikis can see interruptions in the human vitality field and right them to their characteristic condition of reverberation.

The 7 fundamental vitality focuses of the human body are known as Chakras.

Chakras are crossroads focuses between the soul or soul body and the phsyical body existing in the physical universe.

Interfacing these primary point purposes of the body are meridian focuses.

The human body's meridian framework is exceptionally associated with the lympahtic framework, and hubs in the myridian framework joining chakras frequently associate with lymph hubs in the physical domains.

In the event that you are intrigued as such, please continue to Become a Reiki Master The celestial wellbeing source is a perfect wellbeing data site. Communicated sentiments have not been hypothetically examined by underhandedness government organizations.

The act of reiki has been going ahead as a correlative and option recuperating and the advantages of this practice is about accepting the mending as well as having the capacity to mend others too.

In the event that you need to recuperate others, you can figure out how to turn into a reiki ace and appreciate the considerable advantage of self-mending too. Be that as it may, in taking in the reiki method for recuperating, you must keep taking in the art and you don't simply take in it from any other person, you need to gain from a reiki ace and get the mending vitality that permit you to recuperate others too.

Like a military craftsmanship, the act of reiki has distinctive levels of capability. In the initial couple of phases of taking in the art of reiki, you will be known as a reiki understudy. On the off chance that you have experienced the preparation and the learning of mending others and yourself, you can now turn into a reiki expert. These are reiki understudies who have experienced attunement - that process by which you are prepared and taught by a reiki ace about mending vitality.

In the wake of being a reiki professional, you can in any case proceed onward to the more elevated amount of the reiki expert. It is in this level that you have obtained top to bottom comprehension and information of the specialty including its ideas, impacts and its application too. As reiki expert, you will be permitted to show this recuperating practice to reiki understudies as well.

The ventures on the best way to turn into a reiki expert may not be that simple. Truth be told, you need to experience all the levels of reiki capability and you need to experience the diverse attunement levels. One you get the purported 'expert image,' that is a sign and an affirmation that you effectively came to the most astounding capability level and that is being a reiki expert.

Showing and attunement trainings assume a huge part in an existence of the reiki and in your mission to turn into an expert. Obviously, you need to instruct others to end up specialists and to wind up instructors like you as well. These techniques will help you pick up the encounters and learning of an expert reiki and permit you to pick up top to bottom comprehension of everything about the vitality of mending.

Obviously, being an expert of reiki, you need to have the capacities to show others and the craving to take in more and become all the more profoundly. You must be merciful and cherishing and comprehension to other individuals too.

In figuring out how to turn into a reiki expert, you need to impart to others what you have realized on your way when you were attempting to turn into an expert reiki. You can likewise settle on yourself on how you can apply what you have realized as an expert.

Turning into an expert can be an incredible route for your own and profound development too. This is not just about recuperating others and having the capacity to recuperate yourself, it is additionally about you becoming actually and profoundly.

Might you want to turn into a Reiki expert? Then again, might you NOT want to spend your life reserve funds while arriving at that point? Indeed, you don't need to, you can begin mastering Reiki without burning through hundreds or even a huge number of dollars on some extravagant Reiki expert courses!

I am almost certain that you are as of now mindful of the way that the Reiki is maybe the most emotional mending force known to man. Be that as it may, I am not certain on the off chance that you realized that the mending forces of Reiki lie within you pretty much as you are perusing this message!

That is rectify, the forces of Reiki are within every one of us, you should simply know how to discharge the power of Reiki!

There are truly a couple Reiki expert instructors out there that are charging critical measures of MONEY from their understudies and I can say that by and by I detest that! Reiki shouldn't be about cash, it ought to be about recuperating and making this world simply a tiny bit of a superior spot to live for every one of us.

Probably the most perceived Reiki specialists concur my emotions about those lavish Reiki expert courses and that is maybe one of the reasons why they are currently offering their assistance on the web.

YES, you heard me right. A percentage of the best Reiki experts are putting forth their assistance online for all the men and ladies that wish to ace the considerable forces of Reiki. Maybe the best part is that they are just charging a small amount of the expenses of going to some conventional Reiki course. I am certain that they would really offer their help for nothing out of pocket for you however I get its justifiable that they require some wage too to cover their everyday costs.

Reiki is one of the, if not the most capable recuperating system for all of them. Numerous individuals acquainted with it are pondering that how might they be able to turn into a Reiki expert. Here I will uncover the privileged insights of turning into a Reiki expert without spending all your HARD EARNED MONEY.

The truth of the matter is that the colossal recuperating forces of Reiki as of now lie inside you, they simply need to be stirred. A significant number of the Reiki educators swear for the sake of taking parcels and loads of exceptionally costly Reiki expert educator courses, however they are incorrect! You don't have to burn through many dollars to turn into an individual that can ace these extraordinary mending forces.

There is truly no requirement for anyone looking to ace Reiki to take these courses in light of the fact that the forces are there officially, in that spot inside you, inside every one of us. The main thing that you have to do is to wake those recuperating forces, large portions of the Reiki instructors have effectively conceded that it isn't important to take each one of those costly courses to turn into an expert of Reiki.

A portion of the best Reiki educators have understood that the most straightforward path for the normal individual to learn Reiki is by doing it in their own particular security. This is much why they have created online Reiki expert courses that pretty much anyone can take.

There are three noteworthy favorable circumstances of doing this from the protection you could call your own home. Firstly, it will cost you just a small amount of what it would on the off chance that you did it the conventional way. Also, along these lines you will ace Reiki a ton speedier than you would by taking a course sometimes and thirdly, you will get the opportunity to focus on it 100%, since you have downright significant serenity in the sheltered environment you could call your own home.

Chapter 15: Introduction Totreating Others

Treating others will be covered in-depth in Reiki Level 2 training; however, this introduction is included because you will soon be practicing on family, friends and your fellow Reiki practitioners. You may also be called to apply Reiki in a first aid situation. However, you are firstly being called to nurture yourself and become filled with self-love and compassion. With a regular spiritual practice, your confidence shall rise as you re-discover a higher sense of true worthiness. You are then more adept at holding energetic space for others, be a neutral observer, and trust what unfolds during a healing session.

A treatment may last only a few minutes or it can last for more than an hour, depending on the circumstances and situation at hand. At the onset, begin with shorter, planned sessions. During an emergency, place your hand on or over the affected area for a few minutes. This may be enough to bring the receiver into a calmer state. If you need a longer session, you can begin with the same hand position sequence used for self-treatments.

For easier remembrance, the treating sequence can be separated into three sections:
- Head area
- Front body
- Back areas

Similar to Self-Treatments, hold the positions for 2-5 minutes.

BENEFITS OF GIVING AND RECEIVING REIKI

Both the practitioner and the recipient experience many benefits. It is important to note that, unlike some forms of energy healing, Reiki does not deplete the practitioner of his or her own energy. The practitioner actually shares in the healing qualities of a session and often ends feeling quite invigorated and refreshed. One hour of a Reiki treatment is the equivalent

During an emergency, place your hand on or over the affected area for a few minutes. This may be enough to bring the receiver into a calmer state.

to three or four hours of refreshing sleep. In this way Reiki is a natural form of stress relief. Patients can continue to receive any other form of medical treatment and use Reiki to enhance their body's healing rate. Even a short Reiki treatment may bring the following results:

- Deep relaxation
- Reduced muscle tension
- Stabilization of heart rate and blood pressure
- Strengthening of the body's immune

system
- Increased vitality
- Improved function of circulatory and lymphatic systems

In Reiki Level 2, we will further explore the treatment of others as a practitioner in healing sessions.

THE REIKI SHARE HEALING CIRCLES

When you give Reiki to others, you are also receiving as much as your system requires. This accelerates, enhances and creates a deeper transformation. The Reiki Share Healing Circles are a wonderful way to enrich your process. Prior to Reiki Level training, you are encouraged to first attend the Reiki Shares as a receiver. In time, you can begin participating as a Reiki channel.

A Reiki Share Healing Circle

REIKI HAND POSITIONS AND BENEFITS

In general, you place the hands down the body as in selftreatments with approximately 3-5 minutes spent on each position. Mrs. Takata recommended an additional 30 minutes be given to very depleted and ailing body parts and organs. Again, I pass on this information in the event that you need to work on any family members or friends, and to complement any modality of service you are currently using.

Mrs.Takata recommended an additional 30 minutes be given to very depleted and ailing body parts and organs.

Interact respectfully with the energy and use a simple intention as your Reiki prayer for centering: **"Reiki, flow through me and benefit** (name of individual you are treating)." **"May I be a loving Reiki channel for** (person's name) **to receive and accept for the greatest good of all."**

Please note the physical, emotional and spiritual benefits are the same as explained in the Self-Treatments chapter. A general benefit is listed. I highly recommend the book **Heal Your Body A-Z: The Mental Causes for Physical Illness and the Way to Overcome Them** by Louise Hay for excellent metaphysical details, along with affirmations that apply to each body part.

SCANNING THE ELECTRO-MAGNETIC FIELD

Before performing a complete Reiki treatment, it is a good practice to do a general scan of the recipient's energy field so you can sense areas that need more attention. A scan also introduces your energy field to the recipient's. Scan usually last no more than one minute.

We delve into this topic more deeply in Reiki Level 2. This information is being provided briefly in Level 1 in case you are called to be of service or give relief in an emergency.

Do not apply Reiki until a broken bone is set. Reiki acts quickly and a mal-union may form, causing it to be

reset.

QUICK FIRST AID TIPS

Do not apply Reiki until a broken bone is set. Reiki acts quickly and a mal-union may form, causing it to be reset. Apply Reiki after it has been set. (The energy does penetrate the cast!) In cases of shock, IMMEDIATELY place your hands on the solar plexus and adrenals.

Reiki does not replace medical care. It can be used to complement recovery after surgery.

Reiki is not a substitute for medication. The receiver needs a doctor's (not yours) approval to conclude traditional treatment.

In cases of shock, IMMEDIATELY place your hands on the solar plexus and adrenals. Reiki can reduce the effects of anesthetics. Chemicals are cleared from the body with Reiki.

Be sensible and rely on your intelligence and intuition. Most situations are responsive to Reiki.
BEFORE TREATING
The following sequence of photos are provided to visually assist you with conducting a body scan.
1. Place your palms over

the individual's body.

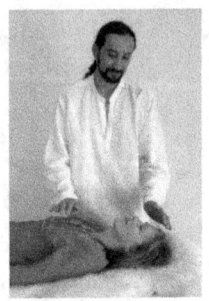

2. Move palms slowly down the body, starting at the head.

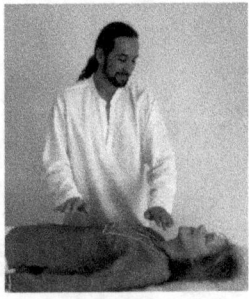

3. Slowly raise and lower your palms as they move down the body.

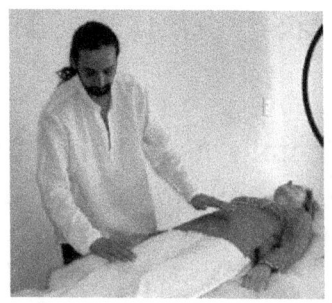

You may sense dips and rises of energy over the body, or hot, cold or vibrating sensations.

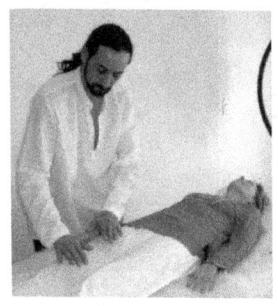

CONCLUDING A TREATMENT
Bring your hands into gassho (prayer pose

and take a deep 4. 5. breath. Mentally give thanks to Reiki for working with you and through you. You can use the following blessing or create your own short prayer :
Feel the "pillowy" sensation of energy above the body as you continue down.

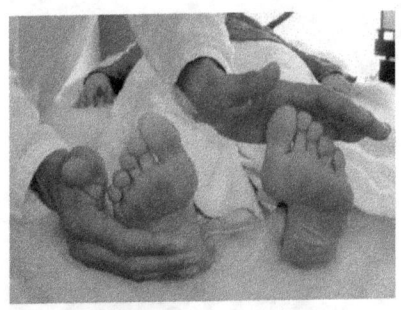

Stay centered and do not mention the possible imbalances in the energy field. This is an indication that an extra dose of Reiki is usually needed.

Finish at the feet. Thank you Reiki for working in and through me. May (person's name) continue to be blessed, healthy, happy and holy.

This blessing can be applied to short or lengthy sessions—even when you are focusing on sending a distance healing (to the best of your ability, by envisioning the receivers subtle energies).

To seal the energy and ground the receiver:

1. Return your hands to the head area and brush the aura by moving your hands and arms in a vertical, circular sweeping motion away from the body. Start at the head and gradually end at the feet. This helps to further clear the auric field.

2. Shake your hands vigorously, sending any released static energies down to Mother Earth.

3. Place one palm on each sole of the foot with the intention of grounding the receiver.

4. Ask the receiver to deeply inhale while they stretch their arms straight back as you gently hold their ankles.

5. Tell the receiver to exhale and hold the breath out. Lightly pull as you hold the ankles. Slightly sway both legs from left to right.

6. Tell the receiver to inhale and relax the arms back to their sides. Gently and slowly release your hold.

7. Stand by the receiver's side as they continue to ground.

8. Help them sit up. Face their backside.

9. Place your left palm at the top of the spine, just under the neck. Place your index and middle fingers on both sides the spine, but do not touch the spinal column.

10. Briskly rub the index and middle fingers down the back THREE TIMES.

11. Return one palm to the top of the spine and place one palm above the tailbone, both resting in place with a gentle pressure. Hold for a few seconds in prayerful contemplation.

12. End with a dedication to seal the healing process, such as the following: **"May you (person's name) be empowered by Reiki ."**
13. Briskly pat their shoulders a few times. Help the receiver off the healing table.
14. Offer the receiver a glass of water and check in with them about the treatment.

15. When alone, wash your hands and arms up to the elbows with cold water to clear and reset your field, eliminating any energy you may have been taken on by over-empathizing, or being too personally attached to the receiver. This is discussed more in-depth in Level 2.

Your 21-Day Cleanse

During the first month of training, you will be assigned a **Reiki Mentor.** Either I or a Reiki Practitioner will be in regular contact with you. This is to help you solidify the teachings, provide support while deepening your new skills, and help you create a solid foundation as you re-enter your environment. You will be journaling your experiences and a summary will be sent to me.

This is a period in which the effects from the attunements are being fully absorbed by your physical and subtle bodies. It is a time of readjustment as all levels of Self assimilate the new energies. Some experience intense emotional releases, while others feel incredible bliss and wonderment. Usually a combination of both is felt. Please honor the process. Be kind to yourself. Do your self-treatments daily during the first 30 days. You are on a grand journey that keeps deepening.

Enjoy the process! Keep smiling and blessing yourself DAILY with the Five Precepts.

Below is a quick-reference guide to consult during your 21-day cleansing journey. Follow it to the best of your abilities. These are only guidelines. Go forth as a bountiful blissful beautiful Reiki Sister or Brother!

1. Journal your observations:

Physical

Emotional

Spiritual

2. Review and practice self-treatment hand positions.

3. Recite the Five Precepts. Before you sleep Upon awakening 4. Attend the Reiki Shares. 5. Meditate on your breath and the flow of Reiki.

Chapter 16: The Human Microcosm And The Taoist Universe

The inner world of the Human Being can be understood from the Yin and Yang polarities and from the energy manifestations of the Five Phases of the Chi Cycle. The Three Pure Forces are reflected in the different planes of existence of the human being. Understanding the human being as a reflection of the Universe can help us understand the delicate balance of the body and the processes of gestation of the disease.

Yin and Yang in The Human Microcosm

In order for the human being to live in harmony, his being must reflect the balance between Yin and Yang that occurs in the Universe. The Yin is to serve as a support for demonstration for the Yang, while the Yang will be responsible for infusing life and ruling the Yin.

If one of the functions prevails to the detriment of the other, harmony is lost and the disease appears. Fortunately, the nature of the Universe causes everything to balance, so that in most cases the disharmonies are minor and the balance is restored by itself naturally, following the laws of the Five Phases.

The Yin and Yang dichotomy manifests itself in the Human Being in different aspects. The balance between blood and energy (function) in an organ is a very important example. The blood is the Yin (matter, cold) while the function is the Yang (movement and heat).

If blood (matter) is scarce, Yin will not retain Yang. This, by its nature, will tend to expand and rise. As a consequence, the body will lose energy and heat. The one you have will be distributed irregularly, becoming congested in the upper parts of the body and being in deficit in the lower parts (the Yang tends to expand and rise).

This situation can produce imbalances at different levels, such as that the more Yin (solid and heavy) parts of the organism will not be able to warm up and become lethargic, while the more Yang (hollow and light) parts will be damaged by the heat itself if it is too. This process is usually evident, especially in internally distributed heat processes. The blood is not able to distribute heat so that the head is heated and the feet and hands are cooled. The heat manifests itself in a pathogenic way throughout the organism because the blood is insufficiently able to distribute and dissipate it. The psyche is triggered, emotions are out of control and the person suffers from hyperactivity, anxiety, lack of concentration, etc.

When energy is deficient, the matter becomes inert, Yang does not give life or rule the Yin. The body lacks movement, it stagnates. The liquids stop flowing correctly and accumulations of substances that cannot be transported to their place occur edema, hypertension, excessive sweating, incontinence of various types, etc. The functions of the body decline. Tissues cannot be fed, repaired or purified. The heat stagnates in the places of its production because the liquids do not circulate. The person lives this state as decay, fatigue, and apathy.

When there is no balance between matter and energy, the Human Being is not in harmony and the disease appears. Yin and Yang are also reflected within the organism at the level of organs and viscera. Traditional Chinese Medicine considers twelve bioenergetic units, six yang, and six yin. The six yin bioenergetic units fulfill construction and administration functions, while the six yang units fulfill functions related to the environment (collection and disposal), transport and storage.

These bioenergetic units manifest themselves in acupuncture meridians. Yin bioenergetic units feed and control a specific organ, using it to perform their functions on a physical level. Yang units have a viscera associated in the same way. The yin and yang bioenergetic units work in complementary pairs. Each unit associated with an organ generates its own type of Chi from the extracted from the Celestial Chi, Telluric, but above all Cosmic. This Chi produced by each pair of bioenergetic units is called Qi_1. The Qi is manufactured and managed by the yin energy unit. The yang unit is responsible for obtaining the raw material for its preparation and eliminating the remaining materials.

Each of the Qi feeds and controls the organs and viscera on which it depends, in addition to certain tissues, psychic areas, and functions of the organism. The operation of each energy unit must maintain the balance between Yin and Yang. When this is not the case, the elaboration of the Qi in which it participates is affected.

If an energy unit becomes more Yang, the Qi made by it will be more Yang and all the parts of the person dependent on this Qi will become more or less more Yang. The same will happen when one of the bioenergetic units becomes too Yin.

In the universe, nothing is isolated, and the internal bioenergetic units of the Human Being are no different. In the following sections, we will see that each pair of bioenergetic units affects the other couples in several ways so that a Yin-Yang imbalance in one of the units implies a global imbalance.

Five Phases of Energy in the Human Microcosm

As stated in the previous section, we have six pairs of bioenergetic units that are responsible for transforming the Chi acquired from the environment to transform it into Qi. This is the correspondence in pairs of the twelve human bioenergetic units:

Organ (Yin)   Viscera (Yang)

Produces and administers Digests and transports

Heart Small intestine

Master Heart Triple Warmer

Spleen-Pancreas Stomach

Lung Large intestine

KidneyBladder

LiverGallbladder

These units are denominated by the name of the organ or the physical viscera with which they are associated. Two of these bioenergetic units, the Master of Heart and the Triple Heater, manifest in their corresponding acupuncture meridians but do not have an organ or a physical viscera. The Master of Heart is a mesh of Chi that envelops and protects the heart. It has a great relationship with sexuality, human relationships, and emotions and collects and manages the whole of Chi not consumed by the organism. The Triple Heater synchronizes the elaboration functions of the different qualities of Chi in the body.

Note that the spleen and pancreas, two completely separate physical organs, respond to a single energy unit. In the same way, the paired organs (kidneys and lungs) are also associated with a common bioenergetic unit.

Each organ (Ying) produces a specific Qi with the help of its attached viscera. The Master of Heart, which lacks a physical organ, does not produce a specific Qi but manages the remaining Qi from the rest of the bioenergetic units.

Normally, Qi is known by the name of the organ corresponding to the bioenergetic unit responsible for producing and administering it. Thus we will have the Qi of Heart, Spleen-Pancreas, Lung, Kidney, and Liver. In this way, we have five different Qi in the organism, and each of them responds to the characteristics of one of the Five Phases of the Chi Cycle.

The Qi of The Five Phases Of The Cycle

•The Heart Qi is developed by the Heart and Small Intestine energy units. It belongs to the Fire Cycle. There are another pair of bioenergetic units belonging to the Fire Cycle: the Master of Heart (Yin) and the Triple Heater (Yang), but these units are not associated with any organ or viscera and do not produce their own Qi.

•The Qi of Bazopáncreas is produced in the Bazo-pancreas set with the help of the Stomach, always referring to bioenergetic units. It belongs to the Earth Cycle and will possess the Chi properties of that cycle.

•Lung Qi corresponds to the lung and large intestine. Su Chi belongs to the Metal Cycle

•The Kidney Qi depends on the Kidney and Bladder. It is within the Chi of the Water Cycle.

•The Liver Qi is manufactured by the Liver supported by the Gallbladder. Its characteristics correspond to the Wood Cycle.

Each Qi fulfills its general functions within the organism, having certain effects at the level of the body, the processes of Chi, emotions, mind, and soul, always in accordance with the characteristics of the Chi Cycle Phase to which answer back.

In addition, each Qi (microcosm) will respond to environmental stimuli (macrocosm) by affinity, so that the Heart Qi will be influenced by the external Chi of the Fire Cycle, the Spleen-pancreas Qi will be sensitive to the external Chi of the Earth cycle, etc.

The relationships between the different Qi are defined by the relationships between the Chi of the different phases. These relationships allow us to define how an imbalance in an element of the Qi elaboration system affects the rest of the elements. For example, an excess of environmental humidity (macrocosm) will affect the availability of Spleen-pancreas

Qi (microcosm). This belongs to the Earth Cycle, which feeds the Metal Cycle and controls the Water Cycle, so the Kidney (water) and Lung (metal) Qi can be affected.

These reactions of the Qi to the environment give us clues about the need to strengthen the organs responsible for producing one or another type of Qi. Thus, a person very sensitive to heat will have to improve his Heart Qi and a very sensitive to cold his Kidney Qi. As for emotions or qualities, we can apply the same criteria. Someone with difficulty concentrating needs to improve their Spleen-pancreas Qi, a sad person their Lung Qi, etc.

In the same way, the Qi creates the internal climate of the person following the scheme of the macrocosmic Chi. If the Liver Qi is unbalanced, internal "winds" appear causing tics, contractures, acute pains that change places, etc.; if the

Kidney Qi is unbalanced, internal "cold" appears causing emotional coldness, stiffness, lack of vitality and heat, etc.

Thus, a person who has been melancholic since the beginning of autumn, neglected in their chores, with frequent colds, who suffers from constipation, has fluid retention in the extremities and dry dandruff in different areas of the skin gives clear signs of an unbalanced lung Qi.

Chapter 17: The Value Of A Treatment

There is no prescribed exchange for providing a treatment. What is important to keep in mind is that treatment does have value. There always needs to be some exchange. Any exchange will do. It does not have to be monetary.

If clients do not value the treatments you provide, your ability to assist them will be severely hampered. Keeping this in mind when letting people know about your practice. Feel free to inform people that you are a Reiki Practitioner, however offering unsolicited treatments diminishes the value to the client. Clients have to ask for a treatment.

Never beg to help someone that does not really want your help.

Treating yourself

As a Reiki practitioner of any degree you can apply your knowledge towards treating yourself. Any pain or discomfort that you experience is an indication that something is in disharmony. You can treat yourself in the same way as when you treat a client. You can perform overall body treatment or a localized treatment which focuses only on specific areas of discomfort.

You can also take advantage of this to practice your abilities. Get a real sense of what a treatment feels like to a client. Feel free to experiment on yourself. You will be surprised what you can learn doing so.

Now that you have studied the key concepts that a Free Flow Reiki practitioner has to grasp before being granted the level of a First Degree practitioner of Free Flow Reiki, you know about Energy, how it works and how it connects everything together.

You have learnt about body energy systems, how to work with energy, how to prepare for treatment and treating someone.

You have learnt how to use the Free Flow First Degree Symbol, how to effectively connect with your clients while staying protected and how to maximize the success of every treatment you do.

You know the Reiki practitioner code of ethics.

Your journey has begun and you are ready to take your practice to the next level. Practice your skills, treat clients and continue your study towards total self actualization.

I wish you all the best and success with your journey.

Conclusion

Our body is a complex machine, which gets into problem later on, if proper movements and lubrications are not provided in the right manner. Food takes care of the lubrication part and exercise/yoga takes care of the movements.

In our regular life some parts of our body are over used and some rarely. Regular yoga helps in taking care of these parts by giving proper movements.

These basic movements give flexibility and strength to various body parts and helps in building stamina for taking so much of strain, thereby making us ready to take on yoga.

Hope this book was useful in getting an insight to what yoga is and how to start with it. Keep doing yoga daily, stay healthy and happy.

www.ingramcontent.com/pod-product-compliance
Lightning Source LLC
Chambersburg PA
CBHW072013070526
44583CB00015B/1456